Preface

For one reason and another, this little book has been five years in the making. Then when it finally emerges into the light of day, it does so in the middle of a pandemic: a little lantern, we hope, to shed some light in dark times. In here, some 70 people celebrate cold water swimming in Brockwell Park Lido. It has grown extraordinarily in popularity: on the day before the Lido closed for the second lockdown, 700 people swam in 11 degrees. Cold water swimming has a long pedigree here: Sarah Atkinson talks to Betty Freddi about the original Icicles in the 1960s and Guy Wickett tells the tale of the modern, informal Icicles of the past decade.

Appropriately, this is a book to 'dip' into and reading it gives an idea why cold water swimming is so faithfully adhered to. Almost no one says it is about exercise: below 10 degrees, most are swimming lengths in single figures. So what's the attraction?

First, there is the high that comes from immersing yourself in freezing water, a high that, if you are not careful, can tip you into hypothermia. To reach that high without too many shivers is a measure of the challenge that cold water swimming poses every day. You are measuring yourself against nature, against the inexorable cold. To do that daily is a great achievement.

Second, Brockwell Park Lido is a place of community, where friendships and deeper relationships are created, among swimmers, and between swimmers and the wonderful staff—lifeguards, front of house and managers. This is a place rocked by gales of laughter and fed by conversation and encouragement and kindness.

It is a great pleasure to be able to thank so many people who have contributed to the creation of *Waterproof*. First, the contributors themselves, listed at the end of the book— without you, there would be no book. Two people have embellished the book, making it a thing of beauty: Sun Ho, the inspired designer, and Lynda Laird, the principal photographer. They have given *Waterproof* its special look and spirit. I thank other photographers, particularly David Grafton, whose images of the wintry pool are stunning. Andrew Corrigan did the film that inpired the flipbook images at the bottom right of every page. Melanie Mauthner is the second pair of eyes every editor needs: she went over the draft with meticulous care, picking out errors and omissions: it's all the better for her reading.

We were fortunate to have organisations and many individuals who kindly supported this book financially: without your generosity, this project would not have got off the ground. We list your names in gratitude overleaf. In this context, last to thank, but not least, is Phil Whall, who led the successful Kickstarter campaign to raise the £4500 needed to print the book. His energy, unfailing enthusiasm and attention to detail meant we made our target with hours to spare—and only a few extra grey hairs.

Finally, dear reader, you complete the circle by perusing this little book ...

Peter Bradley, editor, *Waterproof*

David Grafton

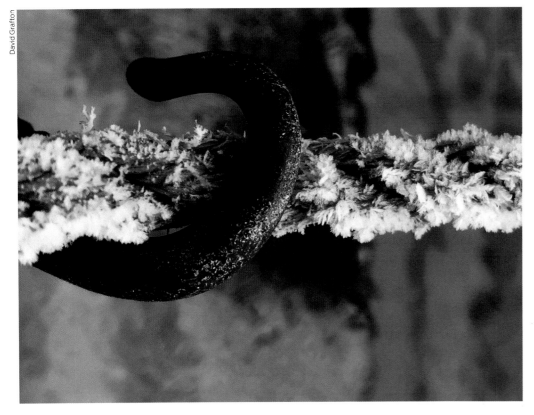

ACKNOWLEDGEMENTS TO THE INDIVIDUAL DONORS

Huge thanks to all who contributed to the successful Kickstarter appeal to raise £4500 to print this book. Here you all are, in alphabetical order:

Tony Allen
Glynn Anderson
Andrew
Eamon James Andrews
Anon
Ant and James
Mechi Arrieta
Marianne Atherton
Sara Atkinson
Alex Balmer
Julie Barlow
Cat Baron
Jonathan Bennett
Jonathan Blake
Debby Boot
Michael Boyle. *Michael led the successful 1993 Friends of Brockwell Park campaign to stop Lambeth Council demolishing the Lido.*
Tom Bradley
Karen Brine
Sam Browne
Adam Bryan
Rosy Byatt
Margaret C
Sarah Cahill
Camila
Alex Carington: *Jon Cowie of Outdoor Swimmer introduced me to winter swimming at Brockwell Lido and it's now my local swim haven*
Linda Casbolt
Paul Casey
Lucy Casson
Juliana Cavaliero
Dee Charnley
Ciaran
Killian Clifford
Deb Conner
Fiona Creagh
Creative Fund by Backerkit
Rosemary Danielian
Dara Óg
Noelene Dasey

Judith De Jong
Rachael Dickens
Chris Durai-Bates
Charlie Eastabrook
Duncan Edwards
Beth Elce
Endymion Road supporters
Rhiannon England
Ed Errington
Denis Fernando
John Finlay. *A donation to thank all of the hard-working people who were part of The Lido Café journey*
Louise Flett
Kerry Fulton
Geraldine
Vanessa Gibbin
Sheila Gilfillan
Paul Gill
David Grafton
Victoria Greenwood
Fiona Grundy
Yolande Hanchen-Elson. *My father Thomas Hanchen is in your book* (Page 56). *He was a regular all year round swimmer at the lido. He has been battling cancer for many years now and very sadly passed away on 1 November 2020. I know he would be so pleased your book is being published.*
Justine Harvey
Debra Hauer
Julia Hawkins
Helen and Peretz
Seb Hepher
Sarah Hibbert
Judith Ish-Horowicz
Miriam Rachel Ish-Horowicz
Fran J
Mike Jackson
Jillian and Paul
Jillian Kay
Tauni Lanier
Yvonne Levy
Lido Mike and Sarah—Streamline Swims
Karen Livesey
Ben Longman
Lucy Luke
James M
Amber Mace
John Mair
Marcus, Katie and Iris

MA Healthcare. *Founder Mark Allen's debut novel,* Life Term, *was published at £12.50 by Colenso Books in March 2021.*
Andy Matheson
Millie
Corinna Mitchell
Laura Morland—*the Lido is a superb gem of this great park, both are loved by so many*
Andy Murray
Craig Naples
Katie Neale
Maureen Ni Fiann
Maisie Olivia
Candida Otton
Patrick and Anna
Jenny Pearce: *Brockwell Lido-er since 2005*
Ian Peate
Alice Playle
Polly
Lesley Preston
Katherine Price
Penny Prodger
Helen Prowse
Emma Pusill
Séamus Rea
Imogen Reid
Clare Reynolds
Julie Reynolds
Michael Richardson
Chris Roberts
Hattie Robinson
Millie Ross
Debs Salmon and Marc Rowland
Tom Shakhli
Julie Smith
Rita Lilian Som
Carole Stagg
Steffan
Matthew Style
Ros Tabor
Stephen Trowell
Laura Vroomen
Carolyn Weniz
Alan and Maureen Whall
Phil Whall
Michael Wharley
Carole Woddis
Marc Woodhead
Marieke Wrigley
Nigel Young

Waterproof

Waterproof, Winter swimmers at Brockwell Park Lido

Editor: Peter Bradley   Swimmer portraits: Lynda Laird, using a Nikon D3   Pool images: David Grafton, using his iPhone
Designed by Sun Ho
Published December 2021 by BLU—Brockwell Lido Users, Brockwell Lido, Dulwich Rd, Herne Hill, London SE24 0PA, UK.
Front cover: Lynda Laird. Back cover: David Grafton
Printed and bound by Rapidity Communications, 235–245 Goswell Road, London, EC1V 7JD, UK. www.rapidity.com

Dedicated to my best friend, Nigel Young, a great swimmer on life's tide. PB

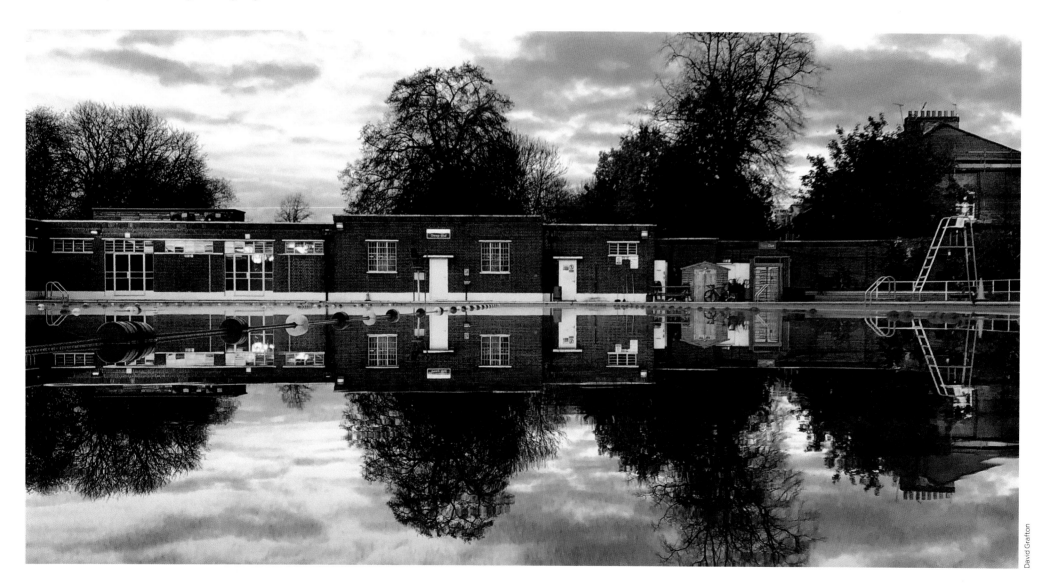

David Grafton

ACKNOWLEDGEMENTS TO THE GROUP AND COMPANY DONORS

Waterproof is supported by:

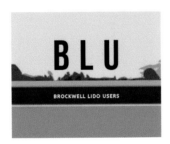

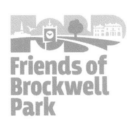

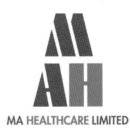

BLU—Brockwell Lido Users
Since 2001, whether you use the pool, gym or classes, we're here so your voice is heard. **www.brockwelllido. com**

Friends of Brockwell Park
Charity working since 1985 to defend and advance the interests of park users. **www.friendsof- brockwellpark.org**

MA Healthcare
Founder Mark Allen's debut novel, *Life Term*, was published at £12.50 by Colenso Books in March 2021. **https:// markallengroup.com**

8 Waterproof

Contents

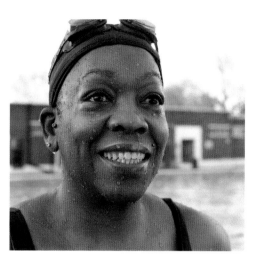 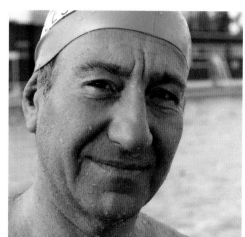 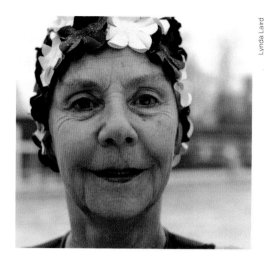
Lynda Laird
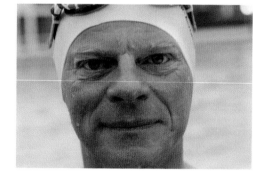
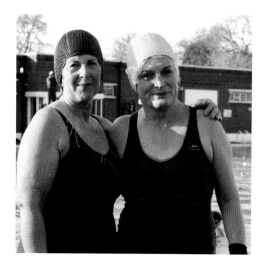

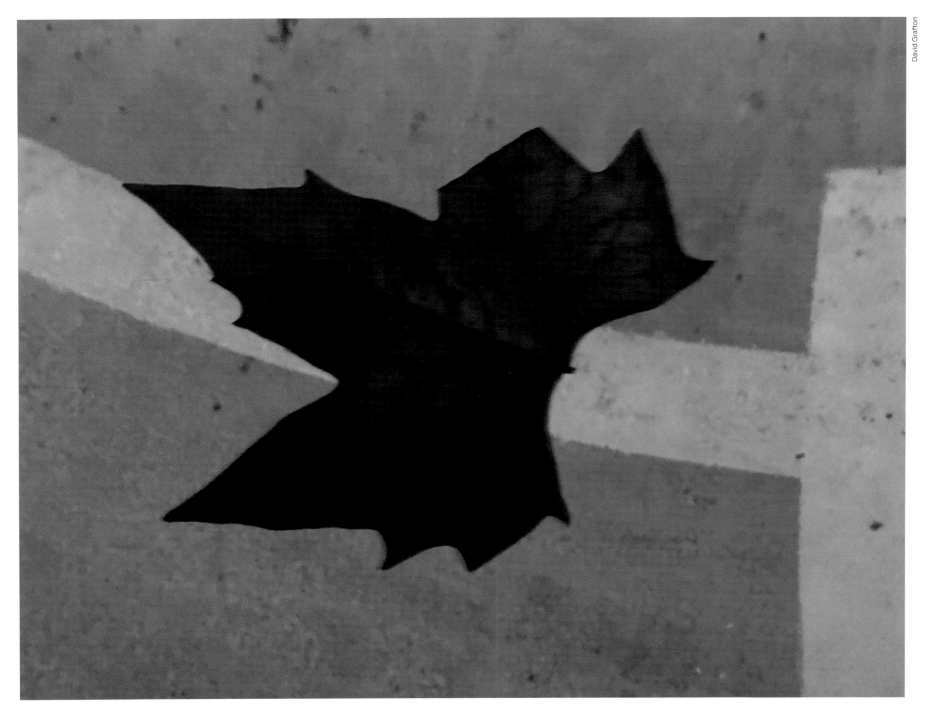

David Grafton

Chapter 1

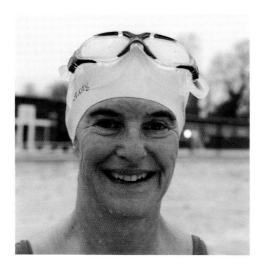

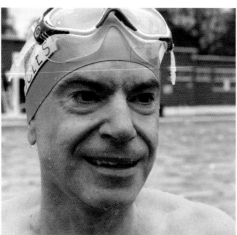

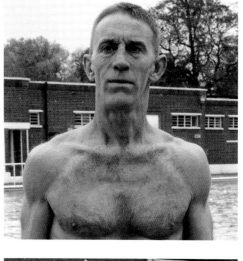

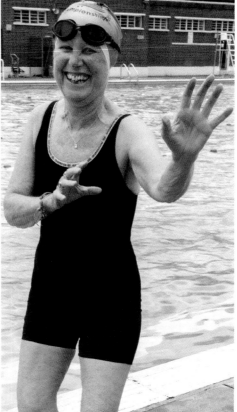

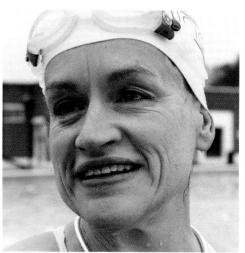

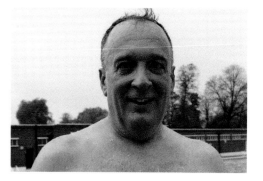

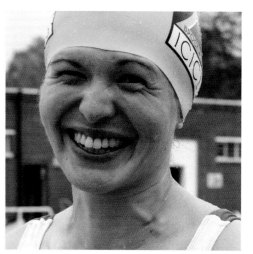

Lynda Laird

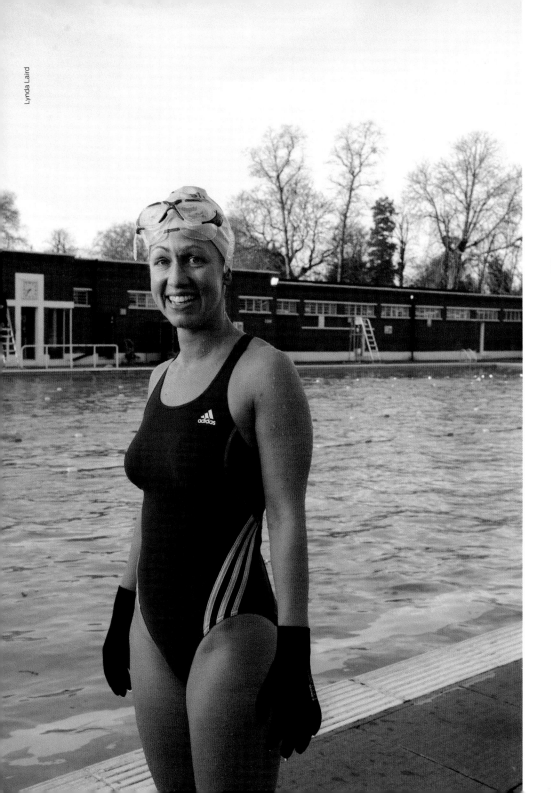

Lisa Bretherick

The lido has changed how I experience the world

The lido has changed how I experience the world.
It has taught me how to feel the world rather than think about it.
It has set me free from the need to achieve.
It's an oasis of calm in a cluttered world.

As I approach I can feel the mist start to lift.
The energy in the changing rooms is infectious.
A spirit of shared experience and genuineness.
The nervous energy kicks in, the questions start in my mind.
Overcome the fear.

Slide into the water and dive.
Peace.
Time slows down.
I see shapes, colours, light and tone.
I feel sharpness, like a hundred needles, but it's not pain,
it's just a feeling.
It's intense, it's pure and it's real.
The water hijacks the senses and focuses the mind.

I am simply experiencing, not trying to achieve or be anything.
I have nothing to hide and no-where better to be.
All my thoughts and anxieties have gone. Clarity.
I'm totally alive.

Everything is okay.

Clare Reynolds

Lido lexicon

to dive in (1): to experience an instant pocket holiday.

to dive in (2): if full of anxieties, fears or worries, clear them by the time one comes to the surface.

head-up breast stroke: the official winter swimming stroke, which allows swimmer to wear woolly hat. Also allows full appreciation of sky and trees, of the changing seasons, and of other swimmers coming, going and chatting. In childhood, was the stroke of safety to keep alert of older siblings approaching to do something dastardly.

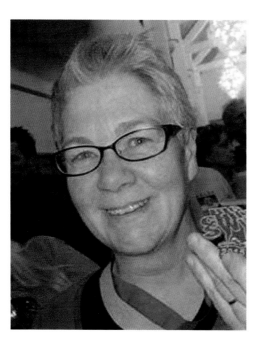

crawl: totally addictive stroke, thought by some (me) to be impossible to do in cold water as the breathing needs to be calm, but now it has become meditative. Allows for the total immersion in the lido blueness and gives entrancing views of reflections and the silvery surface of the water from the underneath. Is a prerequisite for the water calculator and may lead to erroneous belief in superhuman powers of withstanding the cold.

the water calculator: requires no batteries: enter the water with a tricky problem and emerge several lengths later with the solution.

erroneous belief in superhuman powers of withstanding the cold: euphoria develops after too many lengths (how many? impossible to tell), but which persuades the swimmer that they can go on for ever. The swimmer staggers out chilled to the core and will collapse unless carefully warmed up (hot drink, hat, get dry quickly, silk vest), (others may swear by saunas and hot tubs).

synchronised swimming: time travel back to the age of 6, messing about in the pool my Dad had dug, hanging onto his upturned feet as he swam backwards, following bossy older sister's directions to turn somersaults, and laughing enough to risk drowning.

the hunch: the hitched–up shoulders adopted by those unused to cold water, accompanied by shrieks and intakes of breath, who mistakenly think that it's easier to get in slowly. Poor fools, they don't yet know the only glorious way of getting into cold water, to dive in.

a total myth: that one's immune system is better for cold swimming, as I have a totally stinking cold at the mo …

Interview with Betty Freddi
Sara Atkinson

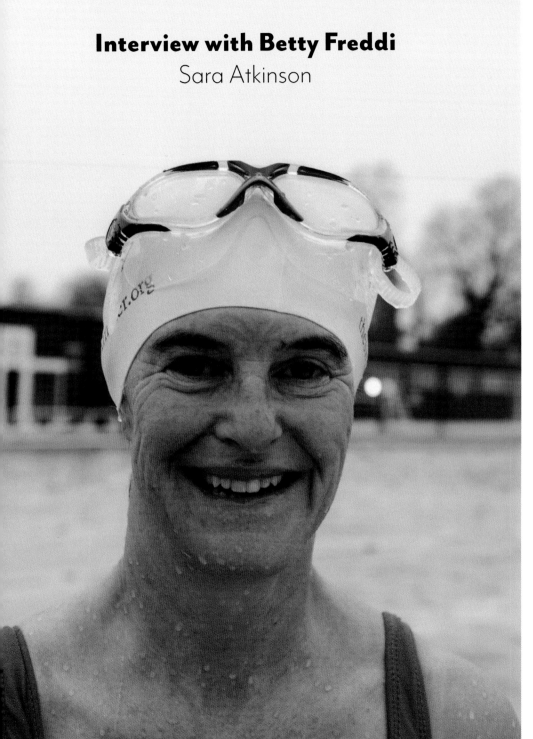

I visited Betty on a lovely April Monday morning after my daily swim. For many years, she has lived in this tall terraced house directly opposite the lido ... it is almost close enough to throw a pebble into the lido. Up the steep steps to the front door and into her warm, neat and tidy front room, I find Betty busy on the phone [discussing paint for the inside of her microwave oven!]. She is a wonderful, straightforward and comfortable woman in her 80s. Her eyes twinkle despite their limitations and her walking around the house is as purposeful as it is unsteady. We sit in the front room and chat about holidays and her daughter, before we drift easily into talking about swimming ...

I asked her about her early swimming memories. 'I grew up in Camberwell and we learnt how to swim at school, but also at Kennington Lido, where I used to go with my brother,' she says. Like many lidos, Kennington Lido and its paddling pool has gone now and in this case is covered up by an all-weather football pitch.

There was a period of time with no swimming. 'During the war,' she says, 'I was evacuated to a place called Hinton St Mary in Dorset. We stayed in a large manor house with cloisters and stables and we had May Day dances. And then after a few years, we came back to a very different life in London, with buzz bombs and rockets. I had learnt shorthand by this time and so, from 1942–45, I took a job in the training section of the Ministry of Works by Lambeth Bridge, where my mother was a cleaner. We used to take the bus home for lunch across Blackfriars Bridge, wondering if the bombs were going to hit us, so I am not really quite sure why we went home for lunch!'

After marrying Bruno, Betty moved to this house on Dulwich Road and it was then that she started swimming at Brockwell Lido. Just as I did when I first moved to Herne Hill, Betty took her young children to the Lido in the summer on warm sunny days. [She tells me of how her daughter Angela had swimming lessons at the Lido as part of a Royal Society for the Prevention of Accidents programme.] There were diving boards and a slide, which have since gone and sadly were not there when I took my children to the Lido. She tells me that there were three diving boards, one high board with two smaller ones either side. 'I remember diving backwards off one of them,' she said. 'How I didn't hit my head, I don't know.' It was the mayor, Johnnie Johnson, who ordered the removal of the boards and the slide in the 1970s for health and safety reasons. Bruno, Betty's husband had said at that time: 'All you can do now is just swim up and down. All the fun has been taken away.' I can't help but agree with him.

Just like me, she tells me that once the children had started to go to school, she took early morning swims and then found herself continuing to swim through the winter. Like now, there were others that swam at the same time, many of them off to work straight after their swim, as I used to do, but perhaps, she says, it wasn't as friendly then as it is now. Most days she said she wondered whether she would be able bear the cold and be able to swim the next day. That is exactly what I used to think and often still do ...

When Brockwell Lido closed for 3 years in the early 1990s, Betty started swimming at Tooting Lido and joined the popular swimming club, became the secretary and edited that Lido's newsletter for 15 years. She shows me some beautifully compiled books of her newsletters containing hundreds of articles, photos, adverts and cartoons, all telling a history of their own. She tells me of the first newsletter in which she wrote about Rosie, a small and slight woman who used to bring nut crackle sweets to share with swimmers on Sundays and used to swim without swimming costume. I was delighted

to hear that costumes were not compulsory then. How wonderful that must have been. I wish we could do that at Brockwell Lido sometimes!

These days, Betty swims regularly in Brockwell Lido in the summer months and particularly enjoys the friendly atmosphere and the helpful lifeguards who walk alongside her as she swims down one side.

'And so, Betty, why do you swim?' I asked. 'I don't know,' she says. 'Perhaps it's a habit first thing in the morning. It's relaxing, it empties my head of worries and it feels good to stretch

out in the water. It's the freedom and expanse.' But we both agree it's terrible when it's full of people.

I wonder to myself if it is the same sort of exhilaration, the same sense of freedom that I and so many others share. Perhaps that's why we love it so much. We certainly share some of the same swimming friends.

'When will you be back in the water?' I asked. 'In May,' she said. Not long now.

On 6 April 2021, Betty Freddi, a legend in both Tooting Bec and Brockwell Park Lidos, died at the age of 93.

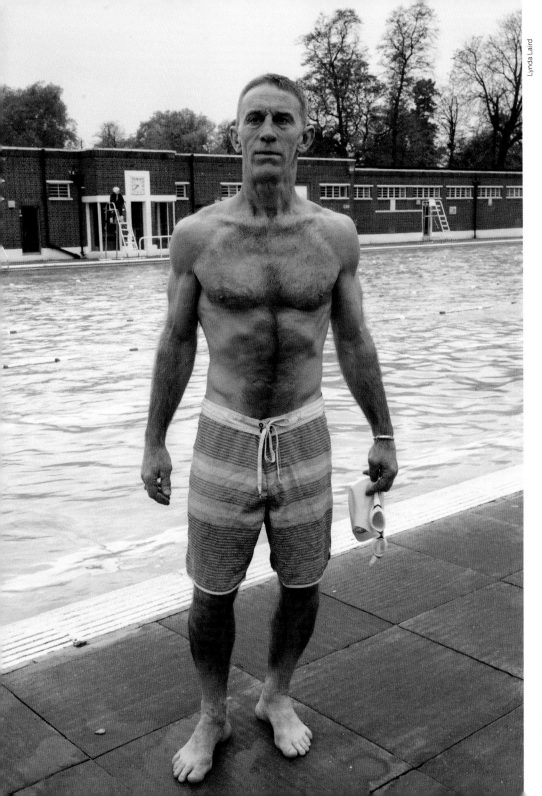

Lynda Laird

Casey McGlue
& ... & ... & ...

I love the fact the Lido is still here
& love the light refraction
when you swim & look back behind you under
the surface, it shimmers
& reflects the water & light

The energy one gets from
cold swimming is also addictive
& great for body & soul

*My only footnote in this book is to pay tribute to Casey, who with Paddy
Considine, from 1994–2002, proved the Lido could be a going concern,
ensuring it survived and flourished. Many thanks, Casey and Paddy. PB.*

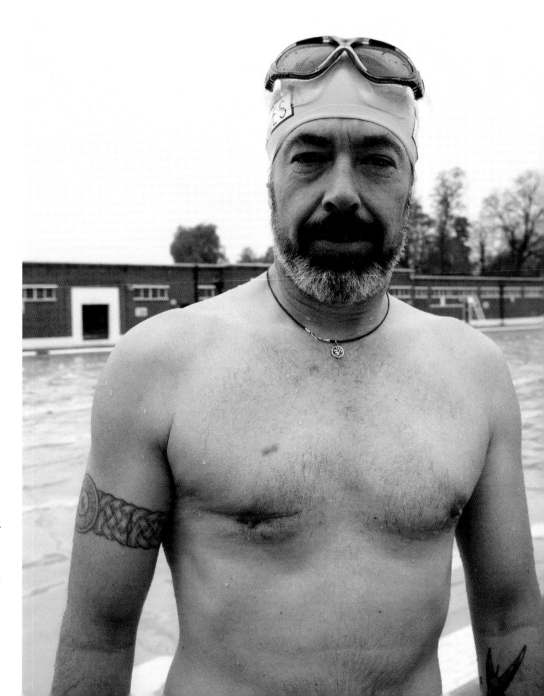

Lynda Laird

Guy Wickett
Friends

A quiet understatement is my Brockwell Lido and it has taken some amount of thought and 'persuasion' to entice me to leave that sanctuary and scribe here ... But that I do and am driven so in an attempt to share my love and addiction of the Lido and the community it serves. (Well that and the freezing cold water and my many friends (and unfriends) whom I frequently share a morning coffee with ...)

In the beginning, it was all about the Rec, a natural gravitation to that fine fortress in Brixton. Impact sports injuries dictated swimming and my endorphin addiction was to be fed by the frantically crowded lanes. Soon part of a changing room full of

regulars, who see each other every morning and despite having known each other for years, rarely exchange more than a smiling nod. Rupert the Bear and I had probably been swimming for four years; the first two we nodded, the third we exchanged names and the fourth a coffee, but only after a chance meeting in the Lido. And as the Lido drew us in, we stood shivering in a late September changing room and said to each other. 'This is shite, how can it close for the winter!?' Looking at each other, a voice was heard. 'Somebody has to do something.' And we did.

Swiftly, a campaign was born, which rapidly attracted others. We harangued Fusion's Chairman after the Brockwell Lido Users (BLU) AGM. MoominPappa agreed to open for three winter mornings a week, if we could attract swimmers. We had a small gathering poolside at the coffee table, trolls and a princess appeared, then a higher gathering in the Prince Regent (my now fiancée and I's second date), special agents arrived and as if by magic, the Winterswim Group was born. Three days became five, five became seven, we evolved into a second reincarnation of the famous 1950s Brockwell Icicles, we were driven to tweet, bought rubber hats. We even invented the Great British Cakeoff and began swimming the winter.

I shall even confess to purchasing a wetsuit in that first year, although I am relieved to declare it only lasted a week—beastly smelly thing, a floatation device taking away all delicious cold sensation and filling with wee—yuk. I can admit I wasn't sure if I could actually swim a winter and was really driven by the desire for exercise, well, and to allow me to consume more cake. Cold water quickly became the drug and if I didn't start my morning with a swim I could barely function. But as the temperatures dropped, other more powerful forces took hold. Yes, the singleminded focus on the sensations of the body, yes, the sun on your face at the deep end turn, yes, the luring azure blue, yesss ... the November 'bite' or the euphoric thrill as you shiver, dashing and grinning for that post-swim train to work. Yes, to all of that, but far far more. Friends. Well, to be precise, cake and coffee with real friends.

And to be more exact, more friends than I remember having ever before, dwarves, goblins, Princes, long shanks, wizards and fairies, hairy fairies (an eccentric and eclectic mix) and not only friends but best friends, people you share your life with, through happiness, sadness, deaths, marriages, genital sores, those you love, those you dislike, new people, old people and equally crazy people ... every single day of the year, year on year—a second family and one so special that frequently you cut short that ever delicious swim, just to have the briefest of coffees with ...

And that's it.

I may ponder that this is not so new, and perhaps we have found something society has lost? Have we forgotten how this may have existed in every street, a lost café community or long closed pubs, that Spanish café culture or neighbourly cup of tea, now sadly missing from everyday lives? But it is certainly reborn and alive and well in Brockwell Lido. And everyone should have one—but only if you are prepared to brave the early morning glacial moraine and freezing cold waters...

This is my Lido. My friends. Very much my life.

Anonymous

(Names changed to protect the innocent!)

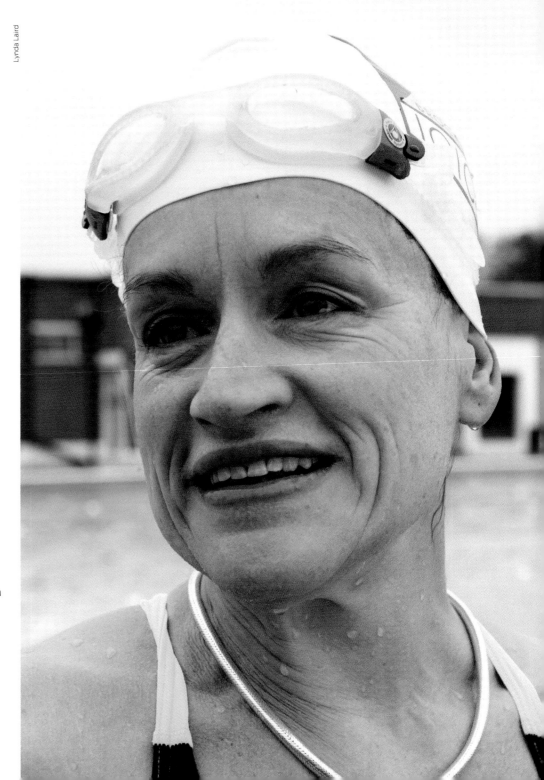

Lynda Laird

Vanessa Gibbin
How brilliant it feels to be alive!

1 November 2016. I made it through to November! And to 11.4 degrees Celsius. Every fraction of a degree lower I feel now. Every day is a new challenge to do something I've never done before. To swim in colder and colder water. It's getting chillier, but I really want to continue.

This morning is an easy day. It's sunny, the park is full of autumn colour. I cycle from home through the park, elation and excitement filling my chest and I want to shout out to everyone about how brilliant it feels to be alive! The autumn leaves are brown, orange, yellow, red. I notice everything as I cycle

through. Swimming makes me live in the moment. It's a perfect exercise in mindfulness. I speed down the hill and approach the lido. My stomach goes and I start to feel nervous—how cold will it feel? How long will I be able to swim today? It's sunny. The sunshine feels gorgeous. I'm dressed head to foot in warm clothes and the winter sun bakes my head.

I arrive at the lido. There's Candy chatting to Stephen. I feel instantly relaxed. I'm part of a cold water swimming community. They're all doing the same thing I am, and they have made me feel very welcome.

I go through the turnstiles and into the changing rooms, past the lido gleaming in the sunshine—it beckons me in with its beautiful blue waters. If I didn't know better, I'd think that it was mid summer and the water was warm. But I do know better!

There's Maureen—she's a counsellor by profession but taking a sabbatical to make a film about a piano. She's never made a film in her life. But that hasn't stopped her. Everyone's trying new things. I say good morning to Anne. She's a fitness instructor with her own local fitness studio. She tells us she's just said goodbye to her childhood home and handed over the keys to the estate agent. A sad moment. She's not swum for a week and is apprehensive about how cold it's going to be. We walk out at the same time—bolstered by taking on the cold water together.

As usual, I walk down the steps into the water while putting my goggles on, then plunge head first and start swimming straight away before sense gets the better of me—and I always exhale as I do. It's bracing. And glorious. Sunshine rippling through as I open my eyes under the water. I love this moment. I feel on top of the world and completely alive. The first two lengths I don't really notice, numbed by the cold, the next two I start feeling cold, by length 7 I feel strong and empowered. As I turn my head to breathe, I see the autumn leaves from the park and surrounding trees. Life is wonderful. By length 9, I feel I could swim and swim forever. Time to get out—the regulars tell me I need to err on the side of caution for the first winter because the high you get from cold water swimming can seduce you into swimming into hypothermia.

As I get out, I can feel the cold air on my skin. But I don't feel cold. Next stop, the sauna by the pool. A small wooden sauna erected specifically for the cold water swimmers, it's like a warm cloak of heat and support. I'm enveloped once again by the community of cold water swimmers and their chat. After 15 minutes, I give in to the nagging sensation that I should be leaving for work and I go out and back to the pool for a quick dip. Amazing. There's the elation and the cold water high again! The changing room is full of swimming chatter—how many lengths, when's the pool opening in full, what time does the café open, how did you feel when you got in, when you got out, what's the weather, gosh how clever Dawn is making swimsuits. A colony of supportive females. I'm showered and dressed in no time and drinking hot coffee from my flask as I prepare to leave the warmth of the cold water swimmers and head to work on my bicycle. Elated. Full of energy and community spirit. I can't believe I've managed another day. I hope I can keep going until December.

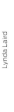

Lynda Laird

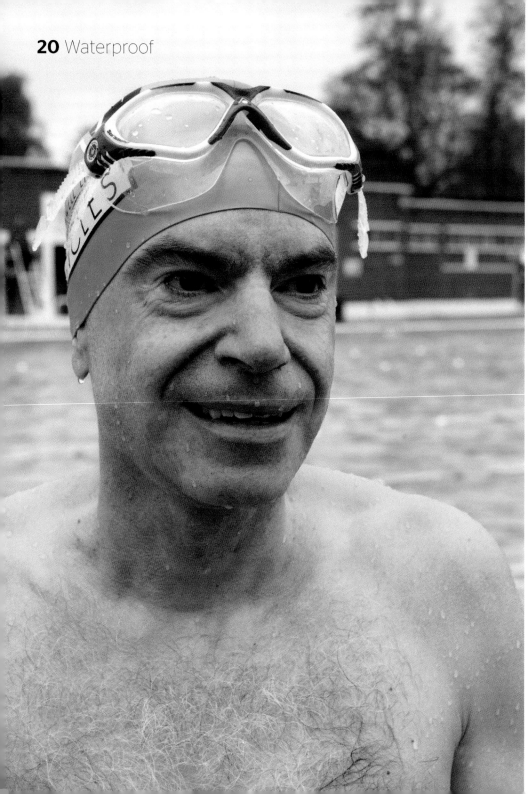

Peter Springett
Want to go cold water swimming at Brockwell Lido? My advice, DON'T!

RESIST the temptation of swimming through crystal-clear water on a bright winter's day.

STEER WELL CLEAR of the super-friendly swimming crew that braves the Lido waters throughout the year.

REFRAIN, whatever you do, from warming yourself up after a chilly swim with the best coffee in London at the Lido Café.

FLEE THE ELEGANT, Grade II-listed 1930s architecture nestling on the eastern edge of beautiful Brockwell Park.

NEVER experience the madness and joy of tip-toeing through snow to a January dip.

AVERT your eyes from the stunning sight of the sun reflected and rippling on the bottom of the Lido.

PROTECT yourself from the mind-blowing rush of endorphins as you warm up gently in the poolside sauna.

BLOCK any idea of partaking in surreal changing-room banter that will put a smile on your face for the rest of the day.

ON NO ACCOUNT get up for early splash and watch the sun rise over the pool as you turn around at the deep end to face the light.

And—above all—**AVOID** life-changing, life-long friendships shared between people of all ages, all backgrounds, and all interests.

All clear? I hope so!

Martin Ashworth

This is now, and that's all that matters

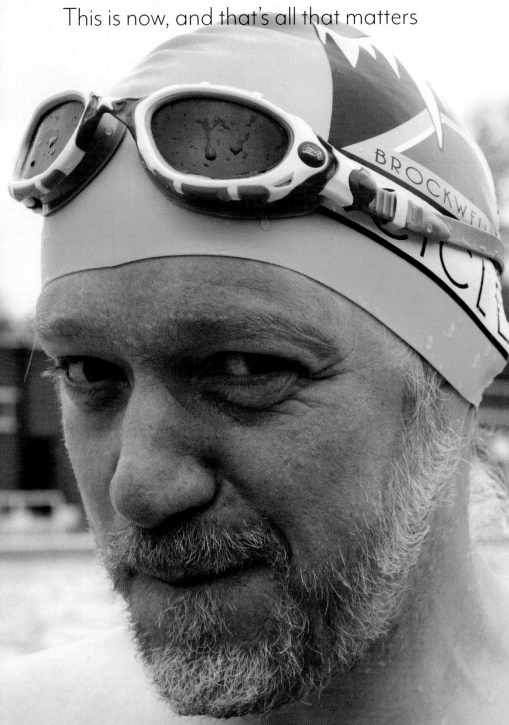

Lynda Laird

There's an annoying chirping sound somewhere ...
It fades, leaving only confusion ...
That noise again, then it's gone ...
The noise ... The alarm ... Bollocks...
My arm reaches out from under the duvet and, with a firm press of a button, the comforting stillness returns, and I slip away, back into the cosy void...

That noise again. For fuck's sake! Arm goes out. Silence. Why did I set the alarm so early?

It must be from when I went swimming yesterday. I'm too tired this morning, so I'm having a day off. My dad used to say something about mind over matter, but it's not like that had anything to with swimming. I'll go tomorrow. It's freezing outside, I can sense it. Just because I always feel better after a swim doesn't mean I'm going right now. After all, it's still dark. I might go later.

My mind is a vague swirl of images and sensations:
Friendly faces, the comforting sound of water lapping, the clarity in the blue.
A gentle breeze on my skin, bright eyes, and the bath of warm sunshine.
The echo of a high-pitched squeal, the wide open sky, the bare trees.
A playful giggle, birds drifting

overhead, and a pair of ducks that landed back last week. Drifting away again ...

That bloody chirping sound ... Up and out of bed. I can't think straight. Aww, look at that ... A packed bag of swimming kit. How thoughtful. Did I do that? And a bike with clothes draped over it, ready to go. I know myself too well ... Slowly leaving the house, closing the door. Looking at the sky, is that a star? Does that mean it's clear? That'll explain why it feels so cold. Pushing the bike towards the road, mounting the bike, and off...

Heading downhill, feet barely in contact with the pedals. Feeling strangely weightless, a touch unsteady. Starting to wake up now. Nobody else about. Stretching a little with each movement on the bike, the air stinging my cheeks as it rushes past. The sun's starting to come up now. There's light in the sky with that pink haze, and a touch of warm yellow, temptingly contradicting the reality of bitter cold.

Into the park now. Trees, grass, and open space. A familiar building. Simple, elegant, single-storey 1930s architecture. Coasting in towards the cluster of bikes, I recognise one. And another. Oh, and another. Looking through the glass doors now. Hints of blue. Nothing specific. Just a vague sense of the colour.

Gently coming to a halt. A familiar face arriving on another bike and a friendly greeting. Feeling part of something now. Anticipation. Something unspoken. Not because it shouldn't be, or for want of trying, but simply because nobody ever seems to have a word for it. Towards the glass doors, the view of the blue becoming clearer. Tangible. Downright stupid.

Through the doors. A gentle hum. An officious receptionist. Another with rather more time on his hands. A view over the water. The peaceful stillness. A clunk of the turnstile. A moment to look out and see an arm reaching from the glacial mirror with effortless grace, stretching forward, and then back into the water. Another …

A reluctant collision of my shoulder with the changing room door. A near-naked body jumps backwards. Shit! Sorry! The figure is friendly, the smile uncertain, one eye looking straight past me, trying to see out to the water. I step back, allow the body to pass, watch it hesitantly hobble out into the cold.

Cautiously looking through the door, the changing room opens up. A sense of familiarity. The smell of damp chlorine. A slight tingle of comfort. The long wooden benches. The same bags in the same spots. The same clothing on the same pegs. The same shoes in the same places on the floor. The showers, the sound of running water, and the echo of a voice, singing opera.

From behind, the sound of the door slamming. A whiff of cold from a shocking pink, wet body staggering past me, a little unsure of its direction as it eagerly homes in on its towel. How was it? – I find myself asking. Amazing! – comes a slurred response. It's not very convincing. I should know better than to ask. Colder than yesterday, apparently. This I can believe.

I find my empty peg and slowly undress. I'm already wearing my swimming kit, having learnt a long time ago how absent-minded I can be in a morning, and how little dignity there is to be found in wandering around outside in wet underwear.
The earplugs go in, and a silicone hat stretches over my head. It's wonky, and a bugger to straighten up, as it drags across my hair. The second hat, even more of a challenge as it sticks to the first in all the wrong places, but I slowly flatten it down and manoeuvre it into place. The goggles go on, and I position them onto my forehead.

I walk towards the full-length, extra-wide mirror, faced with a sight I don't need at this time of the morning. Out through the door of the changing room, the same experience in reverse this time as another uncertain figure steps backwards to let me pass. Instinctively, I take a step in reverse. I'm in no rush, but the polite voice encourages me on through. Turning right, and out into the open air …

There's a light breeze, but it's got a chill. I'm next-to-naked, the floor is cold, hard, pointy and it stings on the soles of my feet. To the left, on the wall behind me, is The Board, a white plastic sheet with the names of the lifeguards in marker pen, along with the opening times and, most importantly of all, the temperature. The distant memory of a reassuring voice – Don't look at the numbers…

To my right, I sense someone, and what sounds like gently splashing water, but I daren't look. I wonder why anyone would choose to take a shower outside in the middle of winter. Surely that water's cold. I don't even want to know. Walking out towards the pool, taking in leafless trees silhouetted against the banded mist that hangs in the last of the night sky, a bird flies low above me.

Looking out across the water, I absorb the elegantly gliding heads in The Zone Of Bewilderment. A lifeguard, perched on a silver giraffe, huddles in bright yellow and bold red. Another one, reluctantly surveying the expanse. Someone changing by the benches, a towel draped over the white rails, crisp against the deep green wall of ivy. The decking. Some serious chin scratching went into laying that. Someone sitting at the table, making tea from a flask of hot water, next to a tiffin of homemade muesli. A cake tin, possibly to celebrate someone's birthday, but it could just as easily be that they woke up early with an urge to bake something new and exotic.

The lifeguard looks down with a questioning smile that already knows the answer, and we politely acknowledge each other. Through the potted palms, the seats outside the café are empty – it's too early by far, the white metal lattice still in place – but the idea of being watched makes me conscious of my posture, so I try to stand up straight, and stride in an attempt to convey a sense of purpose, which is almost convincing.

At the far end of the pool now. The deep end. I can never get in at the shallow end. The idea of walking down the steps and slowly wading out into the cold water… How other people do it, I have no idea. Another table and chairs. More rails. More decking. More ivy. Someone drinking from the water fountain. Someone doing a headstand. Someone else pointing excitedly at vapour trails in the sky. A pair run at the water with an eagerness I can't even begin to imagine. Synchronised, they bounce on the glossy white perimeter of the pool and, in a perfectly-timed, graceful arc, they're in. It's impossible not to smile. I laugh and I can see my breath.

Vaguely standing around like I have nothing to do, I take a moment and it lasts forever. The sun now just high enough to break through the trees behind the far wall of the pool. The surface of the water alive, a channel of warm sunlight dancing across it, widening as it approaches, inviting me.

With a stretch of the arms, I take another moment to see who I recognise. Blinded by the sun, I aim for a trajectory. I shuffle right. A bit more. Left a bit, and I tap the goggles into place. With a deep breath, I bend my knees, lean forward and commit. My legs extending, I feel myself flying over the surface, gazing into the pale blue, and I'm in, rushing through the water.

There's no perception of temperature at this stage, just the ferocious turbulence buffeting around me, but I can feel the colours, opening up. Slowing down now, my view starts to look forward and I can see the expanse ahead of me. The pool looks empty as the aquamarine lifts towards the darker, more seductive horizontal band that sits enticingly beneath the undulating mirror as I gently rise to the surface. With a sudden freshness on my face, I take a gasp and it goes straight back out. Shit! Head up! Deep breath! There's water in my goggles. Typical.

With a kick of deep breastroke, my face goes into the water, back up and out again. My mouth is wide open, but I can't breathe. Nothing goes in. What's wrong? At what point should I signal to a lifeguard? My face goes back in, and I glide, gently this time. With my face back out, a burst of air escapes, and another gasp comes in. I stay at the surface and take a moment, treading water with a touch of the egg-beater. Using a slower, softer stroke, I put my face back in the water. This time I notice it. My face freezes and I'm not breathing out. Lifting back up to the surface, I decide to tidy up the goggles and settle for a length of head-up breastroke.

Between the short bursts of heavy breath, I hear the low chatter of the lifeguards. Nobody else is making a sound. Why am I the only one having trouble breathing? I'm not sure whether I actually feel cold as such, it's too intense to give it a name, but it's obviously too much for me today. I knew I should have stayed in bed. One length will be enough. Nearing the shallow end, a beaming smile approaches, we exchange pleasantries and I try to look as though I'm fine and I've been here for ages. My feet hang down and start to catch on the bottom of the pool between kicks. I stand and walk the last few metres, reaching out to touch the side so the length will count. I turn and take it all in. Feeling strangely drawn back by a compulsion I'm unable to resist, I wade out for a few metres, absorbing the mood.

A floral hat approaches, and I feel a moment of euphoria so I plunge back in again.
Still doing breastroke, my breathing is starting to settle, so I submerge my face and feel the chill rush across my forehead. A deep breath, a shallow dive, and my face feels strangely fine. I give a sustained burst of forced breath out, which is satisfying. The next stroke from the arms, face up, breathe in, kick, face back in again, and this time it's invigorating. My skin, quite literally all of it, feels electric. Now I can feel the cold. It almost stings, but there's an overwhelming sensation covering my entire body and it feels good. A moment of calm and I glide, eyes wide, more relaxed, and with a moment of clarity.

I can't feel one of my fingers. Well, technically, I suppose I can actually feel it, and it hurts. It's tense, and it certainly won't move. I'm not sure which one it is, but it's somewhere in the middle of my right hand and it's ... well, it's frozen. Don't ignore the warning signs – isn't that what they say? I think I saw someone here who's a doctor. It could be serious this time ... I notice goose bumps on my arms and their futility amuses me, then a bird swoops down overhead, the underside of its wings shimmering with a reflection that only a lido swimmer knows, and all I can do is marvel.

Back at the deep end, looking ahead I see the soft sky, the band of bricks now a warm orange lit by the sun, complementing the stunning blue of the water. Hanging on the rail at the end of the pool, I pause and look around. It's all too much to take in, so I push up on the silver tube and sink down. Down a bit more and ... deep. Deep enough to come to a stop and have a good look around. Now I can't feel my toes. Or I can but, like my fingers, all of them now, they're tense and solid. There's no movement there, just lumps on the ends of my feet. Pushing off from the wall, my skin tingles all over in a way that makes me feel alive like I've never felt. I know I probably thought that yesterday, but this is now, and that's all that matters, or at least all I can comprehend.

Coming back up to the surface, I feel ready to go for some front crawl. Each stroke is longer and more poised than the last and I soon settle into breathing on every third stroke. My body twists as I reach out, and my feet give an involuntary flutter which leaves me a little short of breath, so I switch back to breastroke. Excited, I fill my lungs and do a duck-dive, plunging down, and I start to really see the colours. My goodness, that's blue! My arms go out and I drift. I'm flying. I'm really flying! I'm weightless, and I'm moving! I can see for miles, and the tones are incredible. I have plenty of breath inside and I can drift forever, as the bottom of the pool slowly scrolls by with a dazzling tangled net of rippling white lines that mesmerise me. There's nothing else in the world. Nothing. It's just me. Flying. This … is … amazing …

I do a twirl to hang upside down in the water and suddenly realise that I need to pay attention to other people swimming above me, and I reluctantly surface. Someone catches me up and we swim together, but this is not just any old together. When Brockwell Mermaids swim together, they do a graceful dance of breaststroke, side-stroke, backstroke, crawl … Breastroke, side-stroke, backstroke, crawl … We stop at the shallow end and chat for a while, mainly about how wonderful everything is.

Setting off again, this time with a solid front crawl, I'm really starting to loosen up, properly stretching out, with long, powerful strokes, or at least that's how they feel, bearing in mind that someone once described my stroke as 'languid', and the objective viewpoint is probably more accurate. I'm so lost in it all that I barely notice anything else before I glide towards the wall and take the rail again.

How many lengths is that, then? I'm at the deep end so it must be an even number. I can't remember setting off after three so was that the second one? I feel fantastic, so there's no way that's only two. Is that six? I look at the clock but have no idea what time I got in, so quickly abandon that approach. I did five yesterday so surely I'd know if I'd done six today. That must be four. One more will do either way. The mere fact that I don't know how many I'm on means I should think about stopping, but my face feels unusually fine. Sometimes it just goes completely numb. I'm at that point where I feel like I could go for hours, but I'm already losing count and I feel giddy, so it's probably time to call it a day. I'll go for a lukewarm shower, to leave that lingering shiver reminding me of this for the rest of the morning.

I'm definitely having another dive, though. Grabbing onto the rail, I lift myself out like some sort of Olympic gymnast and position myself on the edge of the pool, then realise that my co-ordination is … Well, for want of a better word, it's fucked. I lean forwards and plop into the water in a way that must surely alert the lifeguards. My muscles are really quite stiff now, and my movement is starting to get restricted. My arms don't go out to full stretch, and my legs are of limited use, but the exhilaration is enough to keep me going for one last burst of crawl, although I decide to scull the last half a length, gazing up at the sky and basking in the sun. I look back and briefly wonder if another length might not be a good idea, then quickly catch myself, and clamber towards the steps.

Emerging from the water, grinning as best I can through a frozen face, and singing something to myself that I've just made up, I slowly stagger back towards the changing rooms. My muscles are tense, my breathing is shallow, but my skin feels alive, as I yank the swimming caps from my head, pull out the earplugs, and gaze around me, aware that this might just be the best I'm going to feel all day.

Approaching the door, I glance at The Board. 4.2°. I wonder if it'll get much lower this year. I swear it felt colder than that. When was that measured? I could take a look at the floating thermometer, but I'm on auto-pilot now, thinking only of my shower. I wander back to the changing rooms to find my towel. The costume spinner hums as the water drips out into the curiously necessary washing-up bowl placed beneath it to catch the output. Someone's standing with the hair-dryer up their jumper, while someone else is making a naked phone call to order their breakfast from the half-open café, and it suddenly feels like home again.

I head into the shower, and make comforting noises that slowly turn into a tune. Someone leans in as they pass on their way out and asks – You staying for coffee …?, and I remember that Brockwell Lido is as much about the people as the swim.

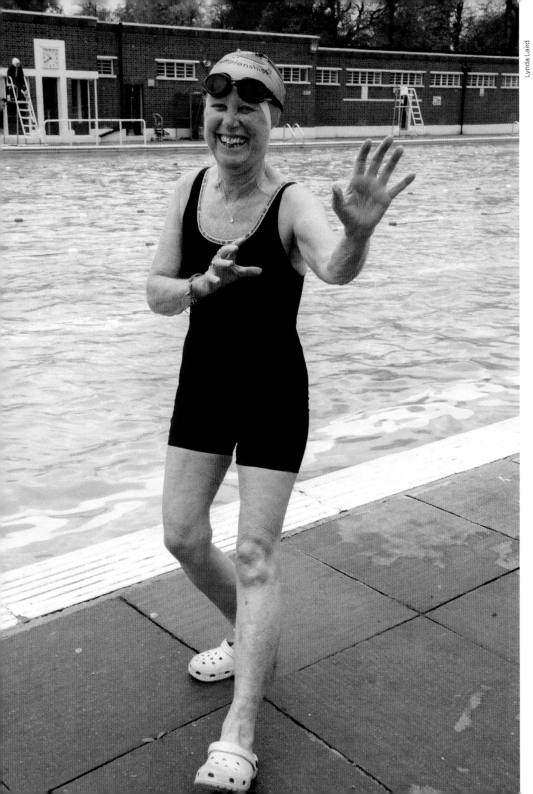

Lynda Laird

Carole Woddis
There's nothing like it

Eyes open. Day starts. Body creaks. Is it a swim day?
Time was when there was no need to ask. Pulse would race. Start the day. Get to the lido, plunge in, or rather step neatly either down the steps or slip noiselessly over the edge.
First contact. Brr. 'No, can't be,' says body. 'What are you doing to me?' But then says, with amazing speed, 'okay, okay, like this'. Now get moving. Breathe in, breathe out, breathe in, breathe out. Get those arms moving, kick the heels. And feel, feel the glide, and then miracle of miracles, senses clock texture of water on skin. And off you go.

There's nothing like it. Colours shimmer. Up come the acquamarines, the velvet blues, melting silvers. Rain, wind or shine, an endless kaleidoscope of colours awaiting you, flashing at you, calming you, teasing you, seldom but occasionally annoying you.
The world is at your feet, or in your eyeline, which ever way you choose to face. Sometimes the cold bites. As the body recedes into stiffness, it resists. It says, 'you may think you think you like this but I'm telling you no lie when I say, I just ain't goin' do this today'.
So, you obey. And sometimes, you lie on your back and you look at the stars, the clouds, the rain pittering down – and you feel for the lifeguards huddled under their umbrellas. And you think, 'This is a luxury, this is a privilege I wouldn't be without for all the tea in China' (and there's an old saying for you!).

But today, it didn't happen. The back wouldn't bend, the limbs wouldn't stretch out, the mind simply wouldn't, couldn't make it.
But there will be other days, you hope, another morning to sense that liquid balm and for a few moments make the world a softer, finer, kinder, more beautiful place.
Roll on tomorrow.

Sunday, 10.15am, September 4 2016

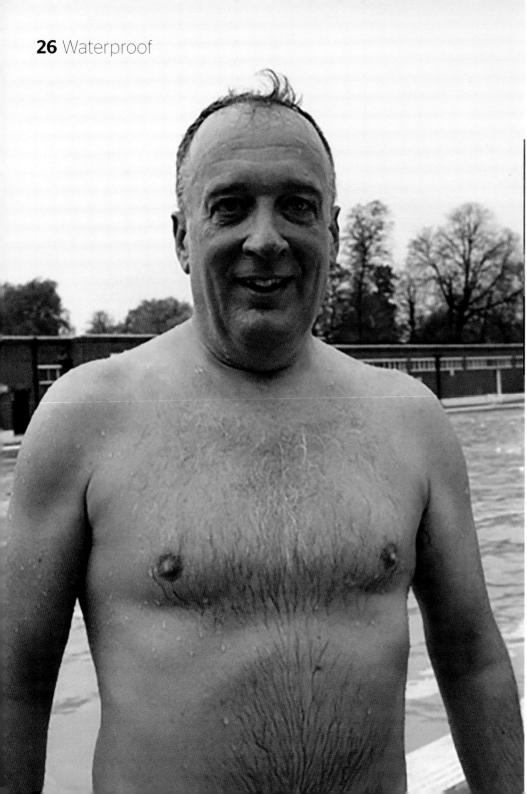

Lynda Laird

Nick Pecorelli
I know it keeps me sane

'You won't believe it, there are people who go swimming in there and it's not even six degrees.' My friend looked aghast when I explained I'm one of them. I am the village idiot, but I know it keeps me sane. And the best moment is the one everyone assumes is the worst: the cold plunge, the dive into the deep when there is frost in the park and the water is still.

I now have reason to celebrate the darkest winters as much as the sunniest summers.

The morning banter lightens the day too. Before the swim, this is based on the equivalent of gallows humour. Our ingrained logic tells us we are putting ourselves through unnecessary pain. But once the chilblains have passed and the immune system reaction kicks in, you get a feeling of euphoria. It's this that is addictive. Then everything is funny and the sound of laughter from the women's changing room magnifies the effect. I am sure the air in there is thinned with helium.

I know that my day will work out fine after this.

The variety of lifestyles and interests of the 'Herne Hill fringe' broadens my hinterland, without me going more than 50 metres in one direction. The personal rituals and eccentricities reassure. The handstand before entry or the handclap after exit. The sequence of goggles and cap placement. The approach to the water or the lane fixation once in. The cake and coffee choice. The hats. The tweets.
I am less ritualistic. I avoid the lanes because I like to vary my speed. I am more of a non-conformist, non conformist. I lament not staying more often for the post-swim natter. Sometimes the ducks join in. They lack lane discipline, but they don't take up locker space. The winter swim is an escape to nature in the heart of the big smoke.
My life is touched by autism, so I know that we must write our own rules. I might be a dog for an hour. We bark together and my son will be happy. Very little of what we know to be true is. We have our own reality and we must embrace it. We are all capable of being village idiots, if only we are prepared to make the effort.

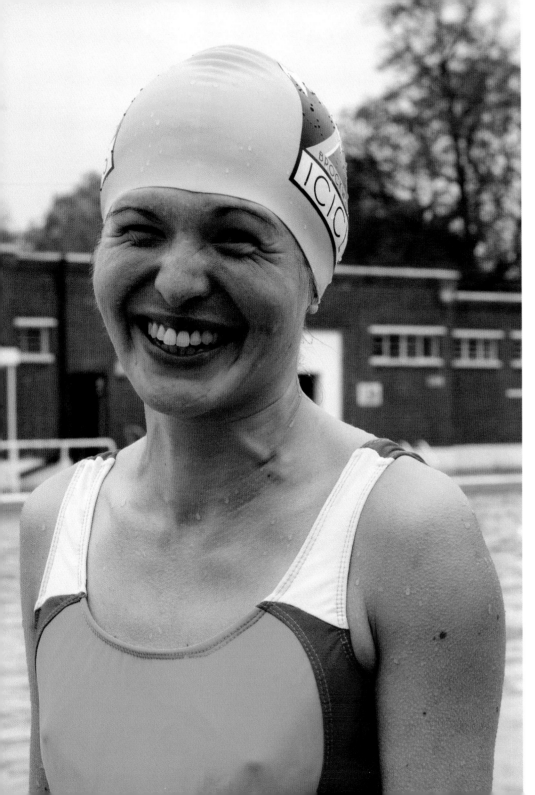

Katie Maguire
A year in the life of a Brockwell Icicle

Autumn

Let us begin in autumn. Your nose is trained to detect the first hint of the cool, leafy smell in the mornings. Exciting times are coming! As the lido temperature drops off below 20 degrees, the crowds recede, thanks be to God, and remaining faces become familiar. But we're still on the extended-hours timetable and so get to enjoy double dips and gorgeous evening swims, the sun peeping over the deep end. Frankly, it does feel nippy getting in, even at 18 degrees. But you're an Icicle! Honour prevents you emitting even the slightest 'eek'. On the way down (going from summer to winter), my favourite temperature is 14 degrees – long enough to comfortably swim for 15–20 minutes, and cold enough for a buzz, that dopey-happy post-swim glow, and – hello! – our old friend, The Shivers.

Winter

Every day is a mini-adventure in winter. By now you recognise everyone coming in and have no qualms shower-sharing with the girls. Hysteria reaches fever pitch in the changing rooms. We all have our own little routines – Sara with the two hairdryers, Helen giving herself a cold blast at the end of her shower, Liz with her carefully calibrated porridge–swim algorithm, me with my peg. Goodness knows what goes on on the boys' side, but they don't half make a racket sometimes. For swims, it's two hats all round, and two swimsuits for some. You hope for ice, but also hope it won't come for weeks on end. Below 10 degrees you get The Fear beforehand, but once you're in, anything 6 degrees and up is HEAVENLY. The lido is clear and crisp; from underwater, everyone looks like they're flying. We could be heroes! Leaves are suspended in your path as if by magic. Colours become brighter and everyone looks beautiful. You love everyone and everything. Basically, we're off our heads on endorphins. We could be heroines!
Under 5 degrees is pretty brutal, I can't lie. Hands and

feet feel like they've been shut in a safe door. You ask yourself why you're doing this and when echo answers 'why?', you keep going anyway. Oh yes, there is of course the coffee and cake at the wonderful café. That must be why.

Spring
After a good few months of proper winter swimming, you're ready for a bit of a reprieve (although I seem to recall snow in March 2013). As the mornings lighten and the air warms, the sense of renewal at the lido is acute. On the way up, my favourite temperature is 8 degrees – it's got it all. Now you're acclimatised, 10 degrees can feel like a luxury, a bath! And the chance to do longer swims in a still-quite-cold and quiet lido seems like

a reward for having run the winter gauntlet unscathed. A few nervous wetsuit swimmers start putting in an appearance around 15 degrees, trying to look nonchalant as they gasp at the cold while we saunter past (OK, I admit I enjoy this bit of schadenfroid (!)). By the beginning of May, temps are usually up and triathlon season is upon us. Uh-oh, this can only herald the start of …

Summer
When Sartre said, 'Hell is other people', I wonder if he had the lido on a summer's day in mind? As Icicles, we are essentially foul-weather swimmers, and I can't deny summer is a challenging time for us. On a hot day, queues stretch over the horizon,

the water goes like mushroom soup (with several hairs in it), and complete strangers start using my peg. I mean really, there are limits. Our group becomes more disparate and we make occasional breaks for freedom at distant lakes and rivers. As I swap swimming costume for bikini, my tan goes into overdrive and I finish the season with a bizarre series of stripes. I think we once worked out the spectrum of emotions brought on by summer, which start with indignation, progress through rage, depression and acceptance, until you reach the final stage, namely, Autumn …

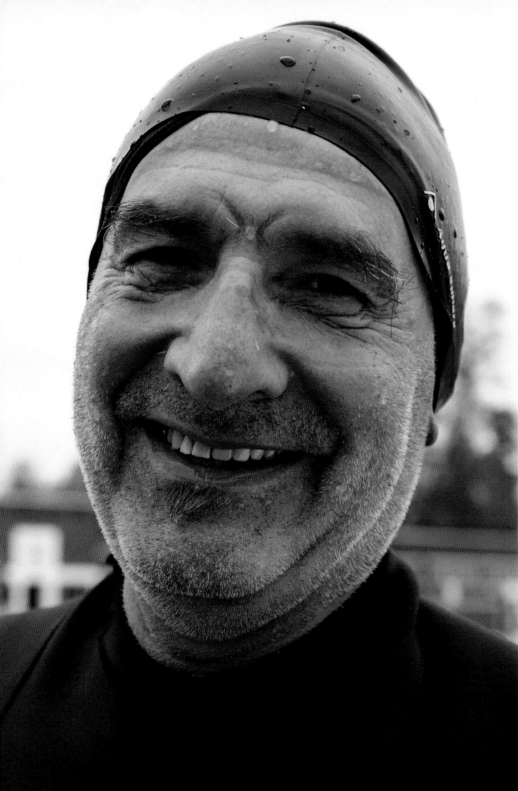

Lynda Laird

Jonathan Blake
This morning it was Golden

I am a novice at cold water swimming, as usually I have departed from Brockwell Lido by the end of September for indoor pools; I like to swim at least one kilometre a day. It is my exercise.

But this year I decided I would continue for as long as I could. To aid me in this task I determined, after many a year of 'pooh-poohing' wetsuits, to invest in a short one and what a difference this has made; we are almost at the end of October and I am still able to swim my kilometre. I am also aided by two swim caps—one's fabric, with a silicone one on top of it—large goggles and ear plugs to keep the cold water at bay.

There is a tiny part of me who feels somewhat a cheat, as I see other swimmers, 'old lags' at the coldwater swimming, who are still only in the swimming trunks, but ...

It is extraordinary how different the actual feel of the water is as one glides through it once the temperature drops to 15 degrees Celsius and below: whereas at a higher temperature it feels silky, now it has this delightful viscose quality as one cuts through with one's strokes, and there is a clarity as one sees the sides and ends of the pool under the water. It is a very visceral experience as one swims. You feel as though you are cutting through the water and parting it.

This morning, which happened to be a particularly beautiful clear and sunny morning, was a special delight, because as the sun is low now when it does eventually catch the water, whereas in summer as it is higher in the sky, the reflection is white light, this morning it was Golden.

The refection on the bottom was flecked with golden yellow glistening patterns and as I swam, especially when doing front crawl or free-style, the droplets off my arm as it left the water were indeed GOLD. It was a delight and revelation.

How long I shall be able to maintain my cold water swimming I do not know, but when and if I can no longer continue it will be with a very heavy heart that I leave. Not only will there be the loss of the delight of this visceral experience, but also the loss of the camaraderie of the other cold water swimmers with whom I share this very special experience.

Chapter 2

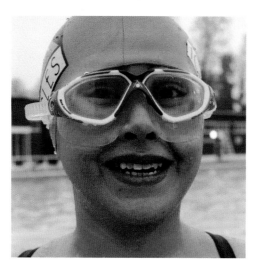
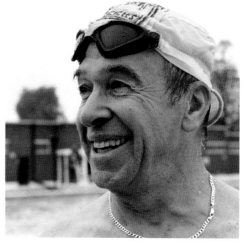
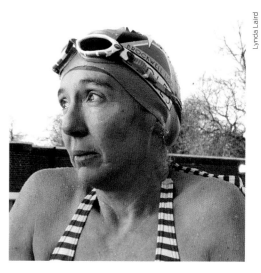
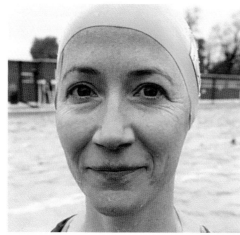
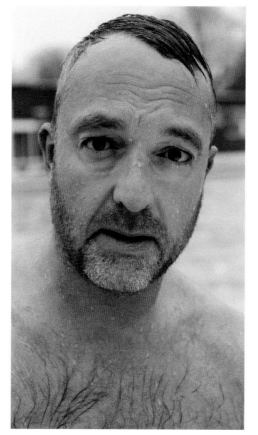
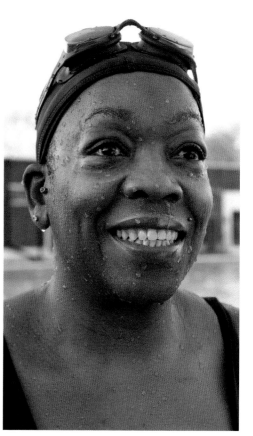

Lynda Laird

Dawn Springett
A Winter's Swim

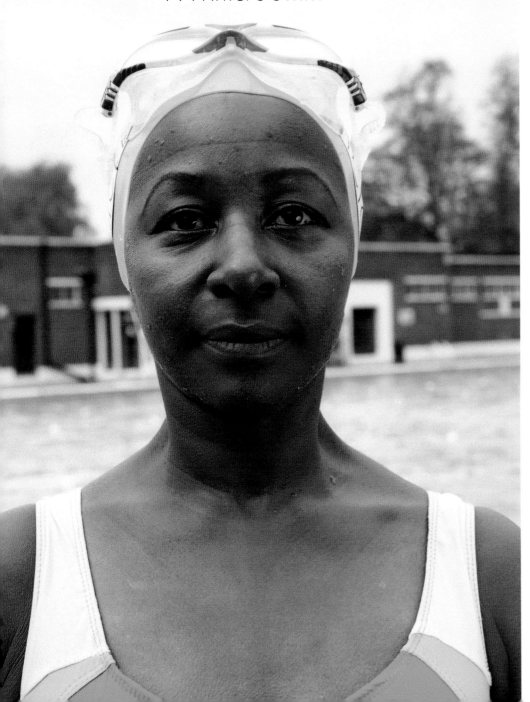

Lynda Laird

It starts with a sharp tingling in my toes,
ascending in a slow crescendo,
lapping against my skin,
my ankles,
my knees,
my thighs,
at which point I just give in
and let go,
immersing myself in the moment,
my heart pounding,
my breath racing,
my breath catching, faltering, spluttering.
I must remember to breathe
In with one stroke,
out with the next,
In, out,
In out,
and when I do, I feel the rush,
the elation,
the high,
the buzz,
all over me now,
the tingling,
as I lose myself,
becoming one with the water,
with the elements,
with the universe,
with peace,
as it finds me at last.
And when I touch the furthest edge
and turn my head,
I'm greeted by a milky sun,
and the day can begin.

Liz Barraclough
Why I don't write about swimming

I don't want to write about cold water swimming. I don't really want to think about it.
The deal with swimming is that I don't have to think about it – it's the place where I come to not think.

Also, I've read enough about swimming. I love hearing what people have to say about swimming. I've read enough beautifully written descriptions of cold-water swimming that I feel I could write one in my sleep: the cold velvety water on your skin, the slight fear and anticipation beforehand, the exhilaration as you realise (again) that you aren't going to die, the euphoria afterwards as the blood rushes through your fingers and toes and you come back to life, the way your lips numb and swell and fizz if you warm up too fast in a hot tub – the same feeling you get when you're really drunk (can you poison yourself with cold the way you can with alcohol?), the feeling that you've done something wonderful with your day before you've even had breakfast, the afterdrop, the shivering, the cake, the friends. I don't think I have anything to add to that.

But anyway, I did try to write something.

I love Brockwell Lido and I swim there almost every morning, through the winter. Thoughts do form in the water – it's mostly just sensation but you can't swim 10 or even 5 lengths without thinking anything, even if it's just noticing the sun on your shoulders, or thinking about your stroke, or wondering if you ought to get out now. Cold water especially seems to invite clarity if you let it, though that might be an illusion.

So I started to let my mind wander while I was swimming, to let myself take note of the way I felt, the half-formed thoughts that would appear and disappear as I swam. And every day when I got to work, I'd take five minutes and try to write down what I could remember. Maybe the smell of bacon from the Lido café, or freshly cut grass in Brockwell Park, or birds flying overhead, or how I felt in the water, like flying in an underwater sky but held down by gravity with no danger of floating away.

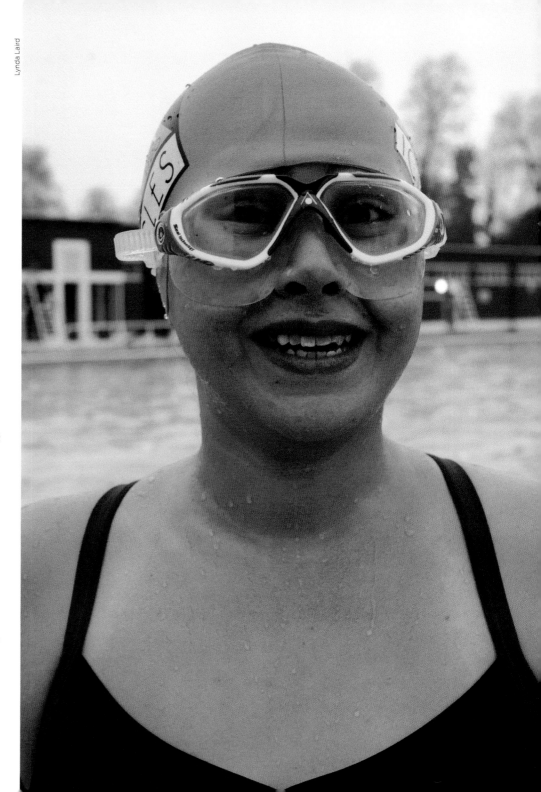

Lynda Laird

Sometimes when I got to work, I'd write more abstract stuff, about why swimming pools were blue, or about other places I've swum in, or the time I painted the walls of my room lido blue and then walked out of a job I didn't much like and had a baby instead. Or about the paradox that swimming is a place (a space? a space in time?) where you can go to be alone, but it's also somewhere you find people.

I've never kept a diary or a journal before, but I suppose that's what I was doing. I found it quite hard to keep the thoughts in my head long enough to get them onto the paper. Sometimes they would seem quite lucid while I was swimming, but by the time I'd changed, had coffee, walked to work and sat down, I couldn't remember it properly. Most of what I wrote was nonsense.

It seemed a better idea to try and write the thoughts down before they could get away, so I began to carry a little notebook and pencil with me. It turns out that writing down how you feel is a bit addictive, and so I jotted things down at random times during the day, whenever I felt something that I thought I ought to remember, or that I might want to read back and try and make sense of later.

Soon, I was writing down all kinds of crap – not every day, but on what I began to think of as a 'bad day', I'd have plenty to put down, flowing out onto the page like water out of a tap. Apparently, I have lots of feelings that I'd never really noticed before. It was a bit overwhelming. I had so much to write down that sometimes it didn't leave as much time as usual to fit in a decent swim.

A few weeks into this little experiment, I found myself writing with complete seriousness, 'The lido is like a prison exercise yard', and walking out of the changing rooms into the park to sit under a tree, drink tea on my own, and think. It was a beautiful morning, the tree was beautiful, all sun-dappled blossoms, with little birds flitting through its branches, and I'm glad I found it.

But it did occur to me that I wasn't enjoying my daily swim quite as much as I used to.

I started to wonder if all those terribly interesting and overwhelming feelings were quite as real as they seemed. Was I bringing out things that had always been there, or was the act of writing feeding on itself, exaggerating

emotions and making them seem more intense? One of the most basic errors in an experiment, where the act of observing starts to affect the outcome.

Around this time, I started trying to take photos again. I don't understand much about cameras, so the way I do this isn't very complicated: I point my phone camera at something that's caught my eye, frame it, press the button and then if I like it I keep it. I like the discipline of trying to fit shapes into a rectangular frame, and I'd describe it more as therapy than photography – it's not much more creative than colouring in.

But I do understand that it's impossible to make a photograph that's a truly accurate description of the world around us or even the view in front of us. The world is three-dimensional, wraps around us, has a feel (of breeze or temperature perhaps), a smell, a sound. The two-dimensional image you create doesn't exist until you make it – it's not the same as what you saw with your eyes. It might be more beautiful, more intense, more emotive, but it isn't the same. The blue you see in front of you isn't the same blue that your camera will create out of light. And the act of choosing what

to photograph affects your depiction of the world – I passed a puddle of vomit on the way to work this morning, I smelt it but I didn't take a picture of it. Another person might have, and it would be part of their view of the world and say more to them than my pictures of shadows and paving slabs.

So I expect it's the same with writing – the act of trying to capture a thought and express it, creates its own entity. Chosen out of the thoughts which pass without being noticed, made bigger and made to seem somehow more definite. Which as long as you are aware of it, isn't necessarily a bad thing. When you learn drawing, you try to draw bigger not smaller, so that you can see your mistakes and how to correct them. And maybe it's the same with feelings – you let them out, make them bigger, have a good look at them in clear light. But feelings are an integral part of you and it's scary to have them made larger, more intense, exaggerated. In order to get on with your life, you need a way of making them smaller again and I worried that I didn't have a way of making them do that.

On top of all this, I had a daytrip planned with

friends, an outing to swim in a river. I was looking forward to the swim itself, which I'd organised, but if I'm completely honest, I wasn't sure if I could stand the company. I'd reached a point where I'd made myself feel so raw and so jarred that I just didn't feel capable of spending a whole day around people. (And these people, I do feel the need to point out, are my lovely swimming friends, the best in all the world, so clearly something had gone a bit wrong.)

Still, it had to be done, and it didn't start badly. An early walk to Brixton tube in fresh air, the kind of journey that gets better as it goes on and the trains and stations get smaller and friendlier and the day gets sunnier. At the other end, we were met at the station by the friendly local swimmer we'd contacted and driven to the river, swapping swimming stories on the way.

There were a few more swimmers there, and the river sparkled in the late morning sun. Wide and tree-lined with a smooth path that meant we could walk a kilometre upstream barefoot, and enough current to mean that swimming back to where we'd started wouldn't be too arduous.

As we walked upstream in the sunshine, I felt calmer and happier than I had done for days and could hardly wait to get in to the water. We climbed down muddy banks, the local swimmers had towbags and understood the river's current and would swim back down with us. The water had a brownish tinge, but was incredibly clean and clear, golden where the light passed through it.

It really seemed like a kind of heaven, sunlight and cold and beautiful golden water with kind, cheerful angels guiding me along so I didn't have to think. (If the people I've described here ever recognise themselves they might find that description hilarious). The swim was even accompanied by an endless peal of church bells from the village church. Without a towbag to hold me back, I could tumble through the water, swimming down and turning somersaults. I'd remembered what I loved about swimming, and felt as though I was returning to a state of grace where I didn't have to try and understand anything, and could just simply experience life again.

Afterwards, we ate cake in the car park. And stood on plastic bags in the car park and rubbed the mud off our feet, and tried to get dressed before our fingers went too numb to do up buttons or hold cups of tea.

I'm an atheist, so I take my spiritual exeriences where I find them, and the parallels with re-birth and baptism are often mentioned with cold water swimming. All I can say is that if you keep swimming, eventually you'll get the swim you need. I've had other outdoor swims where I craved the tension and state of alertness that you only get from swimming alone, but that day it felt right to be looked after.

And when I returned to swim at the Lido, it was as good as it's ever been, we seem to have made friends again. It's beautiful and blue and cold – it even presented me with a sparkling little temperature drop in late April. Even its cloudy grey days are soothing, and I look forward to the company as much as to the swimming. Maybe you need to fall out with an old friend, to remember what you loved about them in the first place.

***

When I'd realised I was keeping a journal, I started to read about why other people did this, what they wanted to gain from it, how – or whether – they kept it under control. Some people keep a journal as a record, others purely as an exercise in writing. For them, the intention isn't to re-read it, just to loosen up their mind or their writing ability, or even to put thoughts down and leave them behind.

The thoughts you have while swimming tend to be like that, they form and flow and float away before you've even got out of the pool. A hot shower and chatter gets rid of them completely So this hasn't really been about swimming, but about what happens when I try too hard to think about swimming.

Is what I've written here an accurate depiction of the past few weeks? Of course not, I've left lots out, and what I've written isn't really accurate anyway. Didn't I explain earlier how impossible it is to do that?

But I had to try and write about something.

Now, if you don't mind, I'm going for a swim.

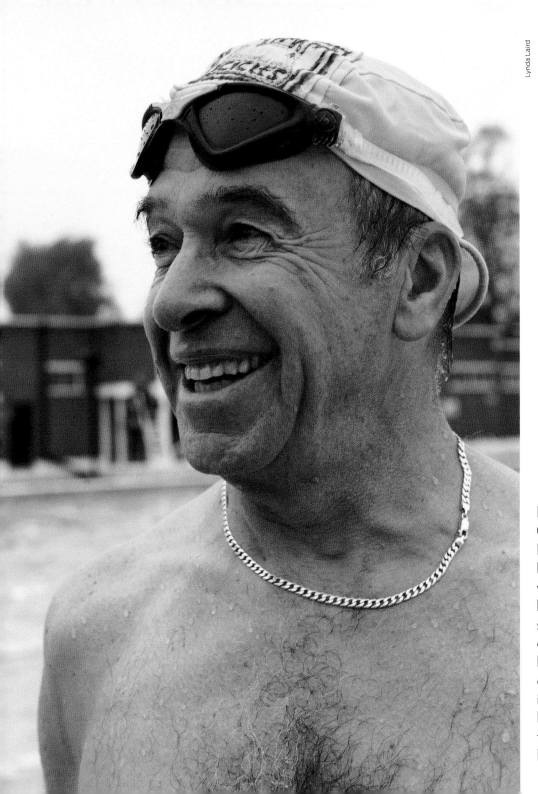

Lynda Laird

Peretz Milstein
I'm water going into water

I learned to swim in the Mediterranean. Our family lived on a kibbutz in Israel, half way between Tel Aviv and Netanya and about eight minutes' walk from the sea. It was quite funny how I learned. I was about 13. My dad stood in the sea up to his shoulder, calling me to him. Being an obedient boy, I walked towards him. I drank quite a lot of sea water in the process, but it was a challenge and I have always liked a challenge. And I learned. Every time I swim in the sea now, it brings back memories of those days in the

kibbutz. I will never forget the walk from the kibbutz to the sea. The sand was so hot I used to pick up vine leaves and put them on my feet. I think it's why my feet today are so tough that I don't feel the cold of Brockwell Lido.

We used to love swimming and the beach, it was the main thing for us as children and teenagers. After work, I'd drive to the beach, we'd picnic by the sea. We'd go naked in the sea, boys and girls; we were teenagers, we didn't care. The

Mediterranean was warm, funnily enough especially at night: the water felt warmer because the night was chillier.

They built a pool in the kibbutz in the 1970s. The lifeguard there was fantastic and gave us all a guide on how to swim. He was a very good teacher. I was amazed that this lifeguard used to watch us all and give hints for each individual on how to improve.

When I was 21, I left Israel and went to the US and then the UK. I met and married Helen and we raised our family and for one reason or another, for more than 30 years, I didn't swim, apart from with the kids in family holidays by the sea in Devon or Cornwall every year. That's life! One reason for lack of swimming in London was that I was not keen on most pools, because of the smell of the chlorine. For several years, Helen did cold water winter swimming in Tooting Bec Lido, but I didn't join her. When she started coming to swim in Brockwell Lido in the winter five years ago, I noticed that you don't smell the chlorine here and that encouraged me to go into the water.

The first time I went into the Lido, I walked in at the shallow end. I could not feel my arm at all, I could not get it to work. So I swam to the first ladder, as best I could. And then I made it to the next ladder and went from ladder to ladder. Gradually, I got used to it. Now the cold doesn't seem to bother me as much as it does other people. At home, for years, I used to take a hot shower and then a cold shower. When I was in the Israeli army, we only had cold showers in the desert. The other guys felt the cold, but it didn't bother me. I never shivered afterwards. I think my internal heating system works differently.

At the end of that first winter season in Brockwell Lido, I felt, I want more of it!

I know for a fact the water is a lot bluer in winter than in summer. We humans are 60 per cent water and because water is part of me, in my mind, it is water going to water, which is why I don't feel the cold. I'm water going into water, it's part of me. There's the joy of being in water when the water is a lot colder. It's more pure. It feels like it's purifying me, coming out of the cold water.

I got my nickname of 'Polar Bear' from Helen, for two reasons. First, the noise of my breathing (before I learned to breathe out through my nose) and second, the way I just slide into the water. I don't make a splash.

Lynda Laird

Fran Juckes
20 lengths at 10 degrees

1. why am i doing this?
2. maybe just do two today
3. this is quite nice
4. four, four, four, four
5. five, five, five, five
6. might only do ten today
7. seven, seven, seven, seven
8. stroke, splash, stroke, splash, breathe. repeat
9. stroke, splash, stroke, splash, breathe. repeat
10. made it! maybe two more
11. breathe, breathe , smooth, smooth, breathe
12. breathe, breathe , smooth, smooth, breathe (this is nice, just another couple)
13. breathe, breathe , smooth, smooth, breathe
14. fourteen, fourteen, fourteen, fourteen,
15. getting chilly, just get to sixteen
16. made it to sixteen, might as well do two more
17. seventeen, seventeen, seventeen, seventeen
18. probably should get out now
19. should I? shouldn't I?
20. committed now, just keep going, faster, faster, touch the end, smile.

20 things I need for winter swimming

1. Bike
2. Lido pass
3. Swim bag
4. Two-piece costume
5. Earplugs
6. Two swim hats
7. Goggles
8. Flip flops
9. Pool
10. Friends
11. Sauna
12. Hot shower
13. Towel
14. Shampoo
15. Brush
16. Face cream
17. Breakfast
18. Spoon
19. Flask of tea
20. Large table to sit round with friends and laugh.

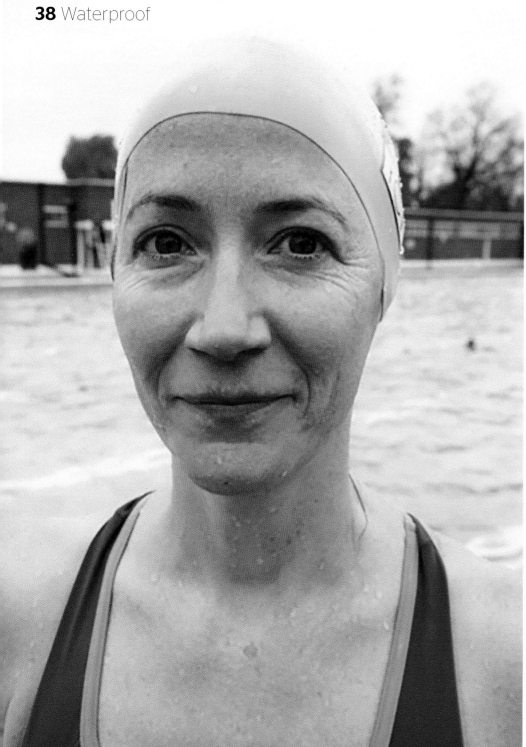

Lynda Laird

Millie Burton
Why do I love cold water swimming?

The colour of the pool—that blue! The sun, or rain or wind, the weather makes it spectacular each time; for me there is nothing like swimming in the open air, under sky, clouds, sun, and sometimes when I'm lucky even the moon to make me feel closer to my animal nature. The red brick, municipal 1930s architecture of the building surrounding the lido creates a frame for the sky, bordered by trees, which in the winter are bare and black. The psychological battle every single time I go, telling myself I'll feel better for it, the thought of getting into that frigid water slowing me down, holding me back, finding excuses not to go, but going despite myself and getting changed into my costume alongside other women, pre-swim doubtful like me or post-swim shivering and high on endorphins—all of us giggling from apprehension or triumph; discussing the finer details of how the water feels or the light looks that particular day, delaying the inevitable walk to the poolside, the climb in, immersion, the first gasping strokes, then reaching the far end and looking back (often blinded by the low sun rising over the wall through the trees and bouncing back up from the surface); feeling every cell in my body alive, my normally sluggish circulation rising to the challenge of keeping this body warm, surviving the intense, delightful shock of the cold. Resting at the deep end and thinking, 'I did it, I can do this!'

I have never ever regretted a cold swim.

Michael Wharley
Those always tempting sapphire waters

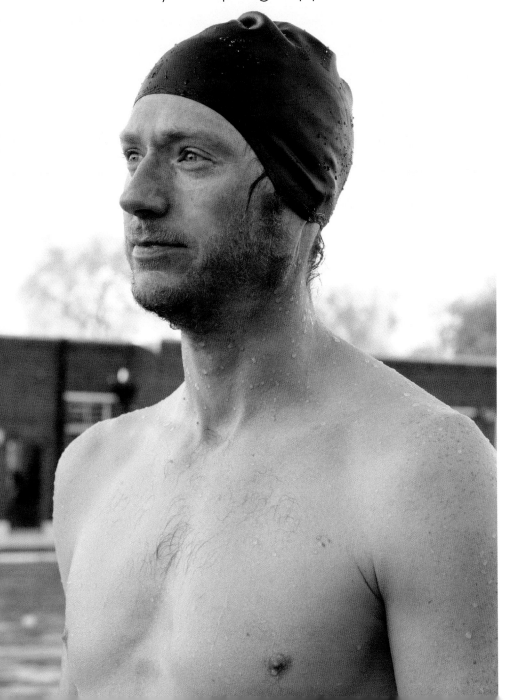

Lynda Laird

It wasn't exactly *Kes*, but the dingy Northern swimming pool our primary school class was taken to for 6 weeks one summer term in 1986 definitely had echoes of a Loach film. Tiny speedos, ingrained dirt, eye-stinging quantities of chlorine and an unreconstructedly bluff approach to teaching that simply suggested, like much in 1980s Hull: sink or swim. More accurately, sink or doggie paddle. I left equipped with no discernible technique, bar an imaginatively inaccurate breast stroke, little affection for any pool and a near-morbid fear of getting my head wet.

Scarcely fertile ground for a profound Lido relationship, but that's what has developed since moving to Herne Hill in 2005. A relationship as deep (at least .75m) as any of the human kind, and as infinitely varied as the endless combinations of light and temperature in the wide open sky above those always tempting, sapphire waters. Not to mention, *in* those waters.

A crisp fraternal backslap on a sharp spring morning, just enough of a crystalled kick in the pool to feel your edges and the benefit. A warm embrace on hot summer 'Brixton Beach' days, the water near-opaque with sluiced-off sun cream and the air almost as thick with the shrieks of overheated children. Then, the shock of rejection, nay betrayal, come October, the good times disappearing

as fast as the mercury drops, single-digit temperatures driving blood to the innermost of bodily recesses, and all but the hardiest indoors.

Yes, the Lido is capricious and demanding, even cruel, but also benign, benevolent and all-welcoming. I suspect we all half-think it is ours alone, delighting in the rare mornings when we swim with only a duck and two lifeguards for company. But really, it is everyone's, and thanks to BLU, that is now inviolably what makes it so central to Brockwell life.

For me, it's where I learned to front crawl (thanks to another Lido institution, Streamline Swims) and where I overcame that irrational fear of getting my head wet. It's where I go to exercise, but also where I go to think. The space, the light, the sky, the blues and whites, the fellow swimmers, even the cold, afford a sort of clarity and a breathing space it seems impossible to find anywhere else in London.

As for that cold—when it is cold, and then it really is properly cold—the anticipation is almost always worse than the reality, but always trumped by the payoff: the radiant post-swim glow—equal parts hyper-stimulated circulation, relief and smugness—that is the very definition of a happy Lido-ite.

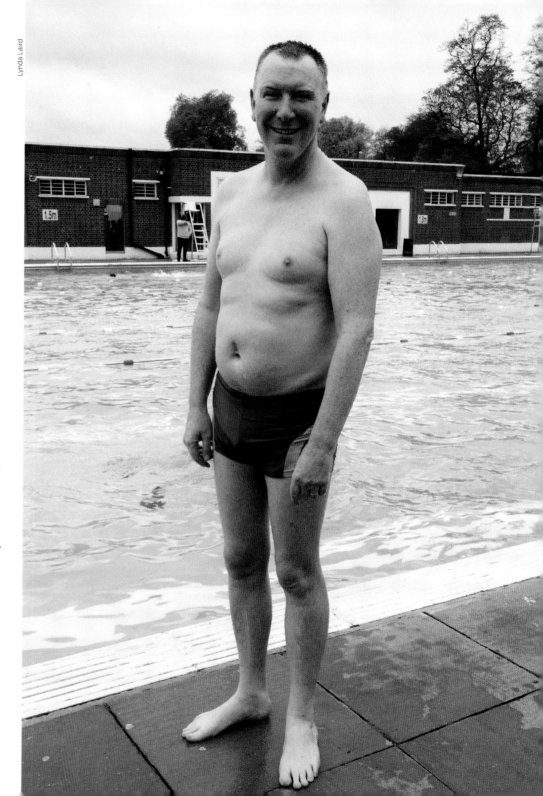

Lynda Laird

Paul Casey
The one constant

I'm not entirely sure about where or indeed whether I officially learned how to swim. I recall being packed off at a tender age to Glenalbyn swimming pool in the Dublin suburbs. I think I just splashed about in armbands and eventually realised that with some self-instilled choreography, my aimless splashing could be transformed into a more structured set of movements —a swim!

Those long hot summers of the late 1970s and early 1980s drew me to the magnificent Blackrock and Dun Laoghaire baths. Seawater-fed, unheated, open-air Victorian delights, they were. Both located adjacent to the railway line and Dublin Bay and

fortunately, both only a quick bike hop from my house.

My newly-acquired taste for the chill of the Irish Sea led me to join my mother in her daily lunchtime sea swims at the picturesque, if pebbly, beaches at Killiney and Whiterock. When her daily district nursing schedule demanded a less lengthy lunch break, we plunged in at the more workaday Seapoint bathing place.

Two weeks each summer saw me holidaying with family friends at Pontoon in County Mayo, the west of Ireland. The holiday home backed right onto the confluence of Loughs Conn and Cullen. Baltic, I feel, aptly describes the bathing temperature of both of these bodies of water, even in midsummer. I was in nearly every day, nonetheless.

Occasional outings from land-locked Pontoon to the beautiful, wide, sandy (and largely empty) Atlantic beaches that pepper the coastlines of Mayo, Galway and Sligo were the cherry on the cold-water swimming cake for me. My appetite for swimming was replaced, in the mid-1980s, by the seemingly more mundane pursuits of studying for exams and job-hunting. By the late 1980s, the bright lights of London town were beckoning and off I went to find them.

A bed on a floor in Crouch End (when nobody knew where that was) and a mind-numbing clerical job at HM Revenue & Customs caused me to pause for thought: there must be more to life than this. I turned back to swimming. At first, overheated, overcrowded municipal indoor pools, then the delights of the newly reopened, deliciously chill, Park Road Lido (originally built in 1929). Directly managed by Haringey Council, its operations were quirky to say the least and even at the height of summer, it closed for an hour at lunchtime, but it was (and still is) a gem. I became a regular and my re-addiction to cold water swimming began.

In 2010, I moved south of the river and as soon as the storage boxes were unpacked, I headed off in search of cold water swimming opportunities. I have been a regular, often daily, summer and winter swimmer at Brockwell Lido ever since. This special place has buoyed me through several challenging life events including a cancer diagnosis. Brockwell Lido and many of its devotees are a big part of my life now and I wouldn't have it any other way.

Fellow winter swimmers wanting to catch-up on the day's news or just tune in to the latest Lido gossip on a winter's morning need do no more than lend an ear to the exchange of discourse between me and my great friend (and BLU committee member), Carolyn Weniz, as we plough through the chill blue water at the pace of a snail. Winter days in London are often dull, sometimes depressingly so, but that is all a distant concern once street clothes are replaced by swimming costumes and swim caps are donned ready for an invigorating immersion and swim. Several lengths later (how many depends on a whole host of things) and we emerge euphoric. Generally eschewing the steamy and tepid environment of the changing rooms, the chatter continues at the poolside benches as street clothes once again replace swimwear and we prepare for the next episode of real life.

Real life for me during the winter of 2015/16 was a seemingly endless series of hospital appointments and cancer treatment regimens. As I was off work at the time, the one constant (which was generally non-negotiable) was my daily swim at Brockwell Lido. I even worked my radiotherapy schedule around the Lido's opening and closing times.

I remember a Scandinavian visitor to the Lido one winter commenting that cold water swimming should be available on prescription, so beneficial had it been to her mental health and sense of wellbeing. I couldn't agree more.

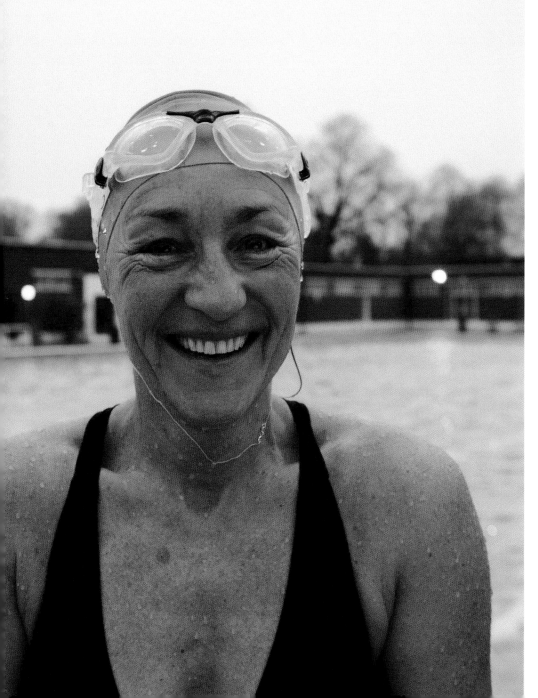

Lynda Laird

Candy Otton
Little did I know what joy

I first stepped inside the hallowed walls of Brockwell Lido about 28 years ago when I moved to Brixton.
Little did I know what joy it would give me for years to come. Throughout my teenage years, I moved around, not really having a base or a so-called 'family home'. Then I fell in love, finally settled in Brixton, and made my own home.

This Lido is special to me for so many reasons. One very important reason being that, one August 24 I left the pool waddling like a duck. The very next day, my lovely Jess arrived in the world. As soon as I could, I took Jess to the Lido. There we played and swam, laughed and swam, snoozed in the sun and swam, met friends and swam, ate cakes and swam, this was just the start. I still swim and still eat cakes and still have the loveliest of friends old and new. Many of the new ones I have met because of the lido and our bond, water.

Brixton Lido opened and closed, was refurbished, changed hands, was drained of its water, so humiliating, but still it held on.

For me, the Lido and swimming is my peace, my haven from the pace and madness of life.

I feel safe within the walls of the lido. Swimming is something just for me, my time.

I am in the moment, it is a rhythm, the seasons pass, the skies constantly changing.

The sun breaks through, the water lights up and greets you with a thousand bright smiles. All I have to do is glide, kick, pull and roll—just pure enjoyment. Then came swimming in cold water—another level altogether. It is exciting, scary, exhilarating and it makes me smile without fail. I sometimes feel butterflies in my stomach anticipating the cold water.

Because of swimming, I have met new friends, swum in waters I would never have dreamt of.
It is a thrill, all my senses are on high alert. A sense of achievement, it is without fail addictive, I love it.

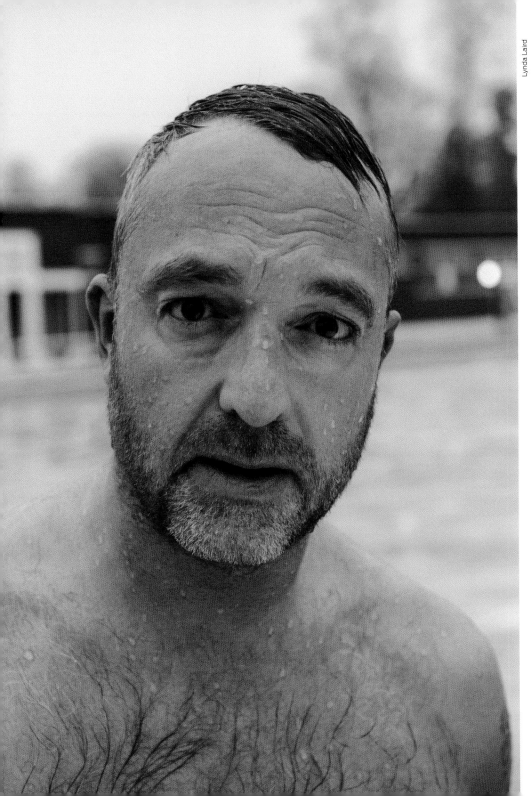

Lynda Laird

Adam Robinson
A shared, almost holy, experience

It's difficult to put into words quite what the lido means to me, and how important is has become. The summer swimming is enjoyable, despite the almost blurred and gluey water, but the autumn and winter months are when the place really comes into its own. The fair-weather swimmers dwindle, along with the shortening of the days. The mornings colder, the fallen leaves brittle under foot as you make your way. In the cold months, every morning is a challenge, from waking in a warm bed in the dark, to the moment you enter the grey, cold abyss. The ritual of putting on a hat and googles drawn out as the time has come once again.

A glance over to the temperature on the wall, a nod to the lifeguard. Then you are in, making your way, savouring the cold clarity of the water and the silence. Counting the lengths, pulling through leaves, seeing the planes overhead, the rare sun rays striking the surface.

The skin prickles against the freezing water, feet and toes aching to be elsewhere, and it's glorious, unique. A shared, almost holy, experience where the routine of life is placed in its corner, as you live and appreciate every moment.

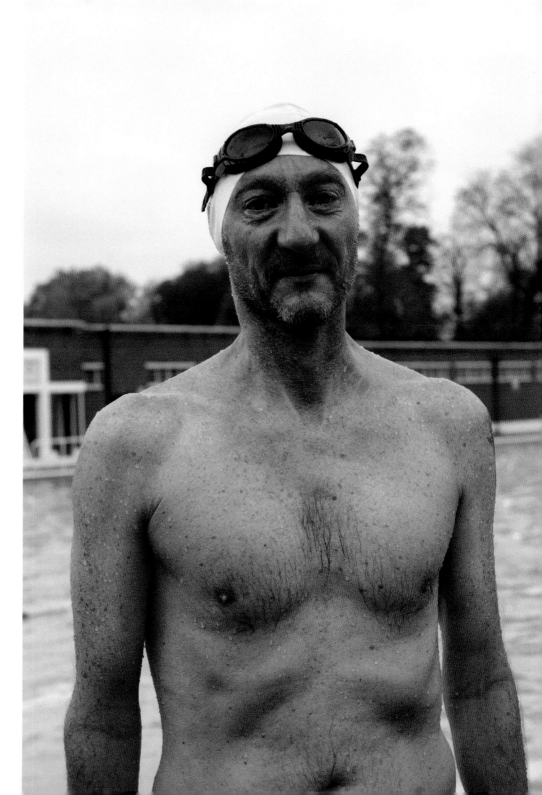

David Grafton
I am a man of water

The cycle through the park the trees the plants the birds the foxes the sounds the smells the light the mist the coldness of the air the excitement the anticipation the butterflies the why do I do this the croissants bagged up ready to eat the view of the emerald city as you speed down the hill the glass doors the reception staff the smiles the lido card all blu and shiny the turnstile the changing room the radiator my radiator the swim towel the goggles the ear plug the trunks the swim hat the mirror the plastic clock the clothes all piled in a heap the friends ... ah the friends ... the endless chat the swim trunk spinner whirring and leaking water the squeals from next door the wosh of the door as you leave the changing room the dithering in the lobby as you stare at the beauty that is the lido the I wonder how cold it is the I don't want to do this the staring at other swimmers their skin pink as they bumble past you the what was that like the encouragement the laughter ... ah the laughter ... the what are you waiting for the are you going in the hopping from one leg to another the are you ready the walk to the door the turning of the handle the springiness of the door the blast of cold air the glance at the temperature on the board the coldness of the concrete the grit scratching your feet the steps the lido café the blu ... ah the blu ... the splashing sounds the squeals the flip flops the clock all square and 30s looking the deep end the warmth of the wall as you stand against it the headstand the stillness ... ah the stillness ... the lido like a mirror in my topsy turvy world the planes in the sky their contrails zig zagging the sky the swim hat pulled tight over the ears the muffled sounds the warmth of the sun on your skin the numbness of your toes

the standing on the edge marveling at the colours dancing in the water the are you ready to dive the hurry up the I'm not ready yet the touching my toes the we must be mad the how many lengths the one two three dive ... ah the dive ... the crispness of the water the bubbles running down your fingers the touching the bottom the gurgling sounds the crystal clear view to the shallow end the coming up for air the glimpse of the trees bare of leaves as you glide through the water the shadows playing tricks with your mind the glittering sun as it bounces on the water the leaves hanging as if in formaldehyde still for eternity the mind emptying the oneness with the water the gurgling chitter chatting the

goggles slowly filling the lifeguards like stone statues watching waiting the graze of the knee the touch of the wall the intake of breath the ... ah that's cold ... the just another length the crystal clear view to the deep end the submerged steps the ducks swollen bellies and webbed feet the white line the rope the plastic bobbles red white and blu the drains plastic clean and shiny the touching the end the warmth of the rail the tingle in the stomach radiating warmth the sun dazzling your eyes confusing your senses the can't feel my feet the beauty ... ah the beauty ... the just another length the tingle in the fingers the ...

I am a man of water ...

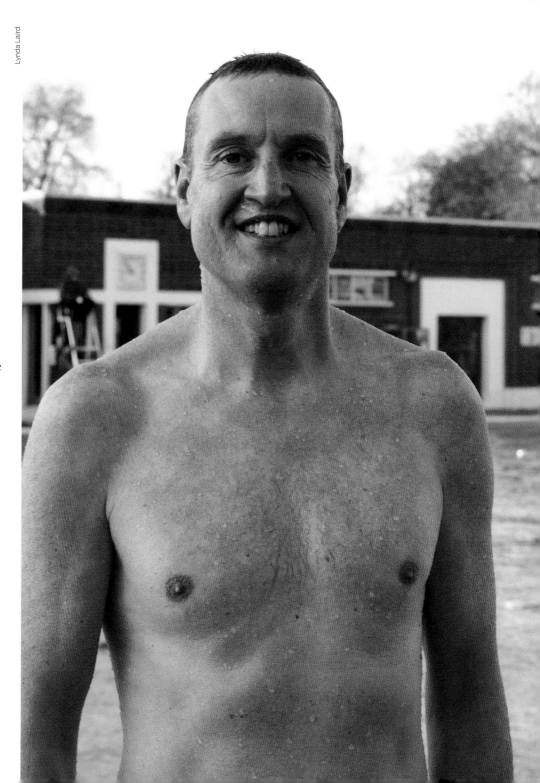

Lynda Laird

Marcus Maguire
I knew from the moment I hit the water I'd found something I was going to do a lot more of

My first proper cold swim was at Parliament Hill Lido's annual 'December dip' four years ago. A good friend of mine, Graham, had done the December dip the year before and raved about it. He tends to rave about everything, though, but there was something about it that really appealed to me. I registered for the event in September during a particularly warm Indian summer. Of course, come December, the temperature had dropped like a stone. When I turned up at Parliament Hill Lido that December day, I remember putting my hand in the water and it actually hurt.

Overcoming fears I might die of shock, I dived into water that was 3 degrees Celsius. I knew from the moment I hit the water I'd found something I was

going to do a lot more of. My body was flooded with endorphins and there was nothing even remotely unpleasant about the experience. I swam two widths of the pool (as per the requirement), got out, raved excitedly, then dived back in to swim another couple of widths. I could barely haul myself out of the water after that, but was pretty much hooked from then on. Brockwell Lido is where I started swimming in cold water regularly. Picking Brockwell Lido was really secondary to another decision I made.

I decided I needed to engage with the world more (meet new people, in other words), so to this end I registered for Park Run. Brockwell Park Run was the nearest to Stockwell where I lived. The first time I did Park Run, I noticed Brockwell Lido situated close to the race finish line. The following week, I brought my swimming things along with me and headed to the lido straight after the run. There at the turnstiles, I bumped into David Grafton (we used to work together as social workers in the West End), who introduced me to Katie. Just as I was thinking, 'she's nice', David whispered in my ear, 'she's got a boyfriend'. Curses!

The initial aim was to swim at least monthly throughout the year, but that soon became weekly, then daily when possible. Four years on, and at the height of summer, I'm hankering for the water temperature to start that inexorable descent into coldness and for the crowds to disappear. I really love Parliament Hill Lido and, dare I say it, might actually prefer it (as a swimming experience) to Brockwell. PH doesn't have the draw of the Icicles, though. I used to swim a lot at the Serpentine too, but got shouted at once by an officious Serpie for swimming outside of the lane boundary. I haven't been back.

I love the water, but wouldn't say I've always been a keen swimmer. I've learned a lot from watching people, seeking advice, having advice thrust upon me, the occasional lesson with Alfonso. I'm probably not so competitive/serious a swimmer as I am

a runner. My main aim when swimming is to relax my body rather than swim fast. For 3 or so years, I combined all three activities by doing triathlons, but I now prefer keeping each activity separate. I love cycling every bit as much as running and swimming, whether commuting, racing, touring, pootling about on Bromptons with Katie (yes, reader, she changed boyfriends).

Irrespective of the water (and ambient) temperature, I always get 'the fear' before swimming. Because I dive in, as opposed to painfully lowering myself in feet first, I'm required to walk the length of the pool from the shallow end to the deep end. A couple of years ago, I made a conscious decision to stop hugging my chest on this fearful walk, as doing so just reinforced any feelings of dread I had.

Arriving at the deep end, I check the time on the Lido clock for no other reason than to delay the inevitable. I dive, and the inevitable gasp in response to the cold translates into the first underwater exhale. 'I'm in,' I think, before surfacing for a breath and starting my swim.

The coldness adds body to the texture of the water, allowing me to pull through it in a way that feels immensely

satisfying. When the water is really cold (under 5 degrees) it feels so cold it's almost hot. Perhaps that's why, when I get out after a swim, my body looks a burnt shade of red.

In the water, though, I'm focused on how my body feels. Even before I've completed the first length, my core starts to warm in response to the energy I'm expending. My hands and feet act as dependable guides informing me how long to spend in the water. Consequently, I never wear gloves or booties. When my hands and feet get painfully cold, then it's time to get out. Bless them, though, this takes time, and until that time my body luxuriates in the coldness.

Being so focused on how my body feels when I'm swimming may be why I'm so unobservant at the same time. Over a coffee afterwards, other swimmers will report having seen glorious light patterns in the water or multi-hued autumnal leaves floating on the surface, neither of which I ever recall. It took me a while to realise that I tend to close my eyes while bilateral breathing (breathing to both sides, left and right), so while I'm swimming, my world is an interior one. After a few lengths, my goggles steam up too, making my underwater world hard to see. I live in my head most of the time.

I don't really see dread and fear as entirely negative, as they're great motivators. I know so many people who experience similar feelings before swimming, in cold water especially. Although, come to think of it, you see people struggling to get into the lido at pretty much any time of year. I don't set out to conquer dread and fear, as much as to ignore it. As soon as I'm in the water, any feelings of dread invariably turn to joy. Cold water swimming is special because it's so joyful. It's all about how it feels. I absolutely love swimming in cold water and don't have any doubts about that at all.

Once out of the water, I get under a hot shower or go to the sauna. That's when the shivers take hold, uncomfortably so if I've swum for too long, which I try not to do. Then it's time for London's finest coffee at the Lido Café, hopefully with cake that one or more of the 'Icicles' have baked and brought in. Inwardly at this point I am aglow, gazing wistfully out at the lido, half wishing I was back in the water.

Yvonne Blondell
because I can

I luv cold water swimming as I feel my mind is focused

I luv cold water swimming as I think it takes training courage and stupidity LOL

I luv cold water swimming as it has helped me move forward from depression

I luv cold water swimming because I can :O)

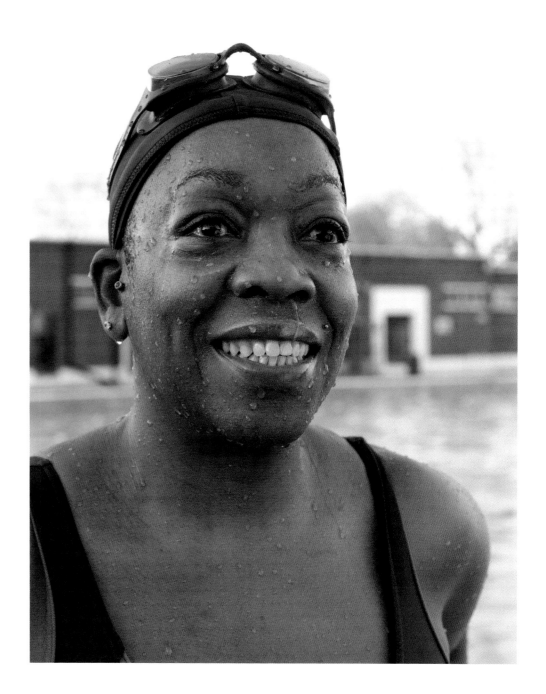

Chapter 3

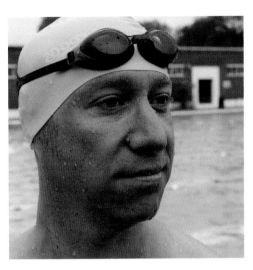
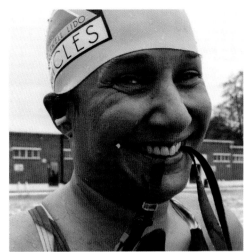
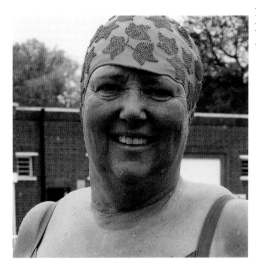
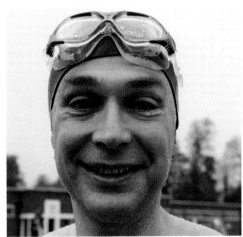
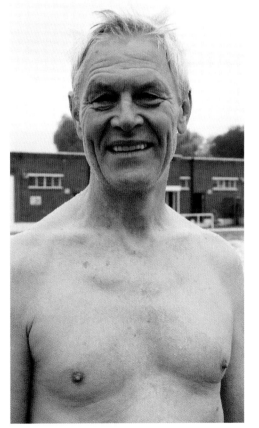
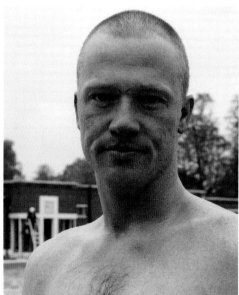

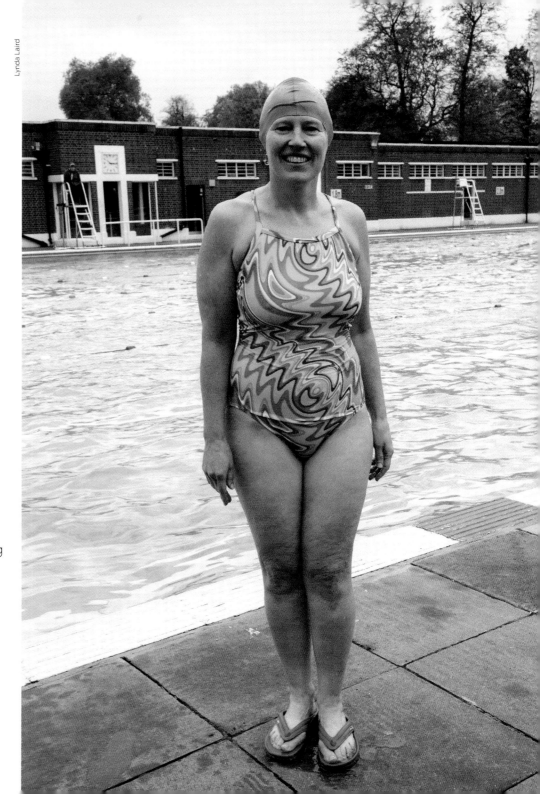

Lynda Laird

Melanie Mauthner
Winter swimming in South London

How I'll miss our temple when I'm
in Russia,
the turquoise water, floating leaves
brushing my face,
the lifeguards in yellow and
Miranda's hedgehog
hat which she bought in
a lingerie shop.

It's our temple with all the
disrobing, gloves,
flip-flops and vaseline. 'Do you wear
ear plugs?'
And who is our god? Rain, wind,
sun, water
we bathe in. There'll be a new temple
in Russia,

there'll be new gods: forest, snow,
steam and lake.
In the shower I wanted to say, I'm going
to Russia soon.
Instead, I asked Miranda about times
and days,

'they haven't decided yet', although
winter swimming
starts next week after the clocks
change. Maybe, in Russia,
I'll sizzle in the banya, my tenses
swirling at midnight.

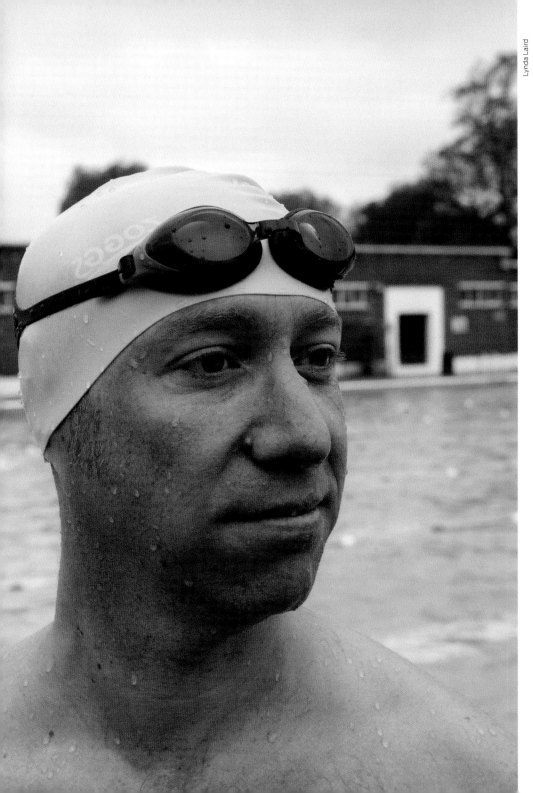

Lynda Laird

Ed Errington
Swimming gives me something back

I learned to swim at dark Thursday evening lessons at Oakleigh Park pool, Whetstone, North London. You'd forget your trunks and have to swim in your pants. My mum has memories of me and my friend regularly crying in the car on the way home. My parents wanted me to learn to swim early, because I'd had an uncle who, aged three or so, had fallen into a lake and drowned. So lessons for five-year-old me were a pragmatic decision as much as anything else. And it was always cold. Cold changing rooms, cold poolside, cold rainy winter air outside. Cold. It obviated any fun of being in water. (A pause while the irony settles).

Then, at secondary school in Nottingham, a swimming teacher, who had been a prisoner in Korea and lost his fingernails to torture, and of whom we were all terrified, barked at me to kick harder in the water. I did, and suddenly found myself accelerating ahead of everyone else. Something had clicked, and without trying very hard, I quickly got good. I joined the school swimming team, and would always do well. But the gala routine was just crappy: the end of day school bell rings, you sit on a bus for an hour down an A road to a nearby school, get changed in the football changing rooms with mud all over the floor,

sit shivering by the side of the pool for a half hour for the sake of a minute and a half zooming through the water, followed by overcooked beans, tepid cardboardy chips, an hour on the bus back, and then homework. Not much fun in that.
So I stopped.

I was about 30 when I started again. I'd moved back to the part of London where I lived when small, and decided to acknowledge the feeling that I ought to do something about the cigarettes and beer. So I went back to the lovely old Swiss Cottage pool where my parents had taken me for fun swims to try and counter the nightmare of Oakleigh Park. I managed about 12 lengths before my legs cramped, and then hobbled/wobbled uncertainly back to the changing room. But I felt good for it, and and tried to make it a routine. A deliberate, forced act of will to go once a week, then twice a week.

Once I'd got to three times a week, I found I started feeling all wrong if I missed a session. And so I was back into it: swimming was great again. We moved house to south London, and Brockwell Lido was on my doorstep.

There are so many things that I love about swimming. It's the only exercise that I have the remotest interest in or ability for. The feel of the water: unlike running (which I hate and which hates me), swimming gives me something back, and it is fantastic. Being outside, turning into the direction of the sun to breathe, and having my vision become drenched with flashes of silver and splash. The joy when realising that the less you do, the more streamlined and better you get. The fact that I find it impossible to hold a coherent idea in my head while swimming: it forces my train of thought to stop, and gives my mind a break. Swimming lets me retreat from responsibility and duty. It's

entirely private. I love that the water will simply take whatever mood I bring to it: I can swim happy, relaxed, angry, or sad, and the exertion involved and the sensation of this textured, invisible stuff moving past me just amplifies the good and drowns the bad. You can primal scream while doing crawl and nobody will know.

There's a wonderful sense of finessing that comes with a long swim. I love the mindfulness that's needed to remember to do all the right things with the correct timing: pointing toes properly, curling fingertips into the very start of the catch, breathing into the trough, getting the two-beat kick working just right with the pull of the arms. There aren't many times in life when I feel like I'm doing something well, on my own terms, but it happens when I swim.

And then there's the brilliant feeling of otherness, that hits every sense.

Cold teeth in mid-winter. The sound of moving water resonating through the extra eardrum of the tight swimming cap. Doing a tumble turn in the lido, facing up while pushing off, my eyes almost overwhelmed by the abstract of the refracted world above the surface zooming past like a waterfall: sky, clouds, trees, buildings, silver water chop. And then, as the sun comes out, looking down at the bottom of the pool, suddenly textured with dancing bright tessellations, and realising that it's about as close to flying as you can get.

I started cold water swimming the first winter the Lido opened for the winter. I dared myself that I would, and asked for contributions towards a wetsuit as an early Christmas present, so that guilt would hold me to my promise. That year it got down just below three degrees in February. There was snow on the side of the pool, and I bumped into ice in my first length. It was like swimming into a broken pane of glass.

One of the most unexpected things about discovering winter swimming was how 'cold' got new meaning. Not in the sense of 'colder than you've ever known' but, rather, in the sense of how it stopped being something simply associated with general discomfort: that anxious, just-want-to-be-warm sensation that came with those first swimming lessons. Instead, the notion of 'cold' opened up completely, revealing a complex and subtle spectrum. Under 14 Celsius, the difference between degrees is really palpable—increasingly so the colder it gets: 4.5 degrees is a world away from 5 degrees.

I recall the real sense of freedom that came with the moment when, acclimatising to the cold for the first time, I realised that I was actually going to be okay in it. It means that you can relax into the water and acknowledge the sensations that the temperature brings (cold water can feel: feathery; lambent; thick; fizzy; hard; nettle-like; hot; and a million other things). The only thing I still find disconcerting is how my heels can start to go numb an hour after I've got out of the cold water.

I love the way that swimming in cold water constitutes a total system reboot. I may feel tired and grumpy before getting in the lido, but when I get out, it's like my soul has been squeegeed. In a good way. And the sensation lasts for hours.

Through swimming at Brockwell, I've made some baby steps towards open water swimming. I did the Dart last year and am doing it again this year, as well as the Bantham Swoosh. I love that they represent personal challenges, but aren't competitive.

The character of open water is totally different to that of the lido, and the way the scenery changes over the route totally offsets the kind of repetitiveness that you'd get swimming inside in a heated, 25m pool. Getting ready for the Dart swim last year, I did some swims along the shore in the sea. That was harder: swell is weird to swim through, and I really don't get along with salt water in my mouth. So I think Brockwell Lido is where I've settled.

The only ritual I have about the lido is, when I'm swimming in a suit, to take it off for the last couple of lengths. This way, I always get a feel of the water on my skin. Apart from that, Brockwell Lido is just a place to relax and treat myself to the otherness of cold water. Swimming in a couple of races in the past few years has confirmed that it's not for me: the idea of people being better at something than others feels increasingly irrelevant,

even though it's all in fun. I don't go for the swimming club kind of thing: I already feel like I belong at the lido, and don't need that ratified by the formality of a named group. For me, the pool is a place where structures, hierarchies, and status get left at the turnstile on the way in. One of the most pleasing things when I started swimming through the winter was that it took almost a full year before I had any idea what any of the other swimmers did in their normal lives. It's as if the absurdity of it all immediately forges an unspoken bond between swimmers. We're just people drawn to the same space, sharing this weird love for getting very cold in water in the middle of winter, and marvelling in how brilliant it feels.

Lynda Laird

Noelene Dasey
Delightfully pointless

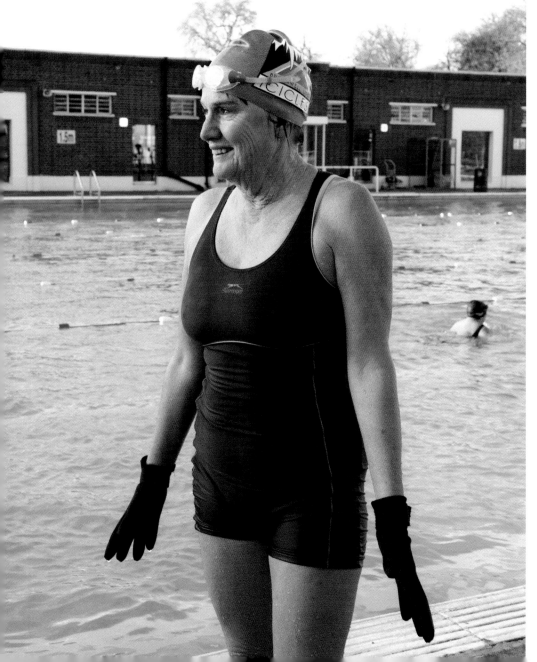

Small, hot, country-town Australia ... The worst of country towns ... Summer holidays stretch from Xmas until February ... youngest of 5 ... I am the really annoying little sister.

Weeks of boredom and blue skies stretch ahead. My mother always ill and away. I feel a bit lost.

It must be around a mile to the pool and it becomes a daily ritual ... zinc cream nose and shoulders ... the really hot walk, cossies and shorts, grubby feet in thongs ... swimming and messing about. Talking, not talking ... it's just passing time.

Fast-forward half a century Brockwell lido ... and I am home again on the wrong side of the world. It's February again ... same blue, cloudless sky ... sun on the water. I am 6 again. Not much swimming, lots of hanging about ... talking, not talking ...

it's just passing time.

At times when I feel lost, I just want to be there. The winter is best ... it's quiet ... the swim is delightfully pointless ... there is no obsession to train, there is no fitness to be had. It is time out of time; big skies and my London family.

This is me ... growing up poolside 1962 (middle of the bench ... aged 2 ... concentrating on the task at hand) with my brothers and sister and cousins. Not much has changed ... Lattes rather than lollies.

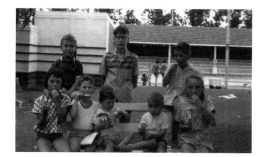

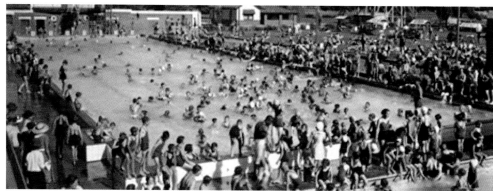

PS The 'New Olympic Pool' in Victoria Park, Dubbo, New South Wales (now the 'Dubbo Aquatic Leisure Centre'), was opened in 1935—a year before the Berlin Olympics and two years before the Lido. The town had a population of around 3500 and within the first 4 days of opening, around 13 600 visits were recorded. This photo is from December 1938. You can just see from the buildings at the end that it is in a very similar style to Brockwell.

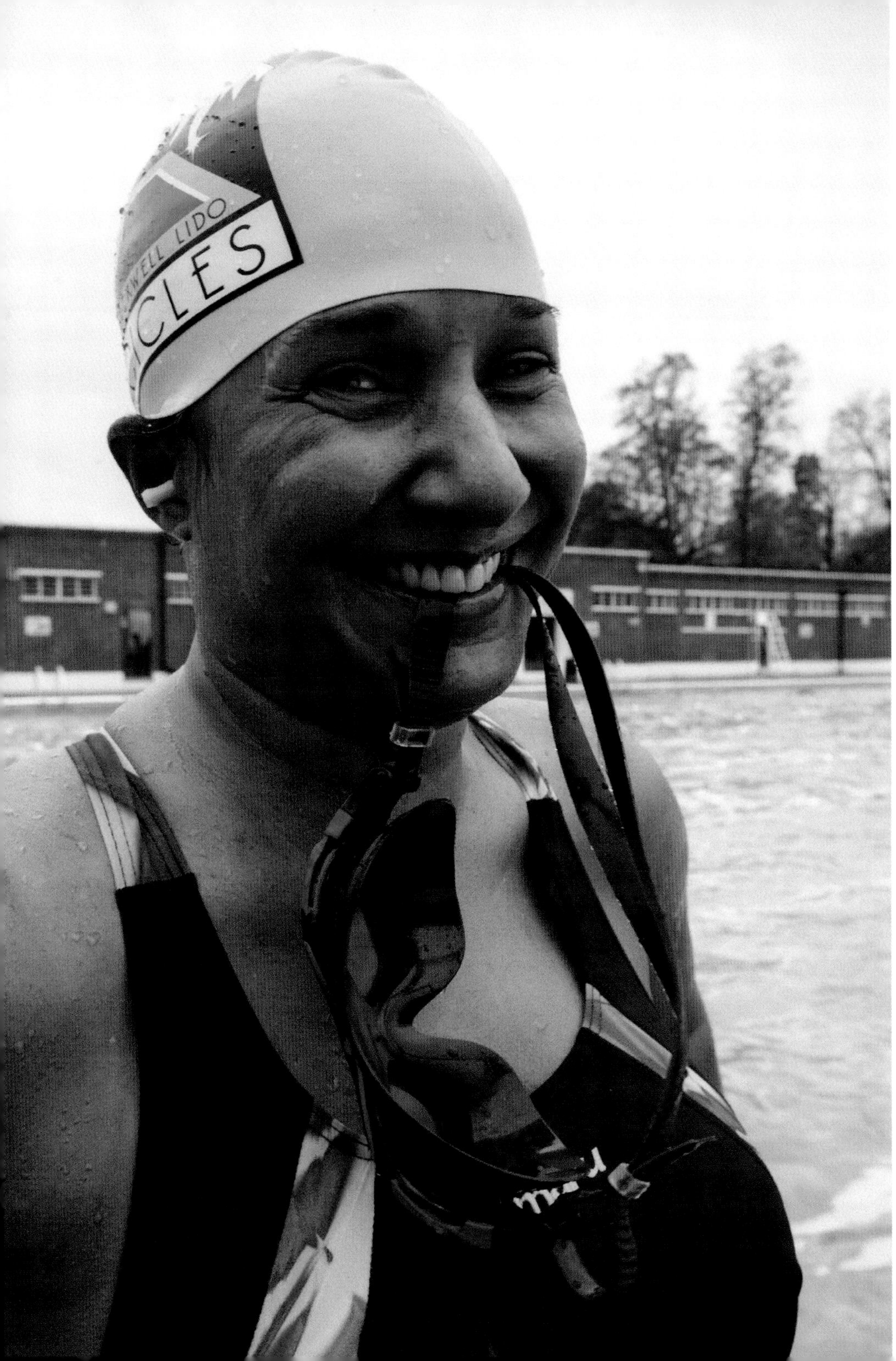

Lynda Laird

Tauni Lanier
Into cold water, splash, gasp

Into cold water, splash, gasp
Needles on the skin
A thought—to stay or swim; swim

Bubbles rising like small globes
Focus; muffled sound
Primordial cold swimming

Clarity of cold water
To swim, onward swim
Take a moment to focus

Why I cold water swim:
by a self-proclaimed *fainéant*

What is there to say? Raise your hand
if you have ever been able to talk
yourself out of something hard ... out
of something easy? Of something that
you did not care about? I bet all of us
would raise our hands on all three. I
view open water swimming (OWS)
in cold water as one way I can have a
caring and thoughtful talk with myself,
and reduce the hand-raising.

I am very convincing ... I can even talk
myself out of something I love.

OWS, especially in the winter, gives me
the scope to test myself—to play with
my willingness to understand the fine
line between anticipation and dread. I
go knowing that the first 50 metres will
be the hardest, that every inch of skin
will prickle with the burning of
cold, knowing that when I get done
with the hard-fought metres, I have
climbed a metaphorical, and at times,
emotional mountain.

[...] knowing that I will have bragging
rights for the day—that I can pick up
the conversation at a moment's notice
with any random person, of any age.

Having a story to tell and cultivating
small pleasures is what keeps me
going—the inability to talk myself out
of embracing swimming in the cold
supports my swagger.

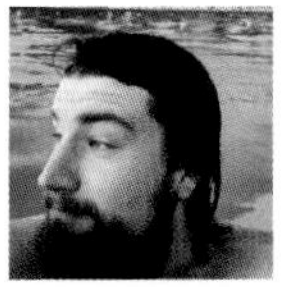

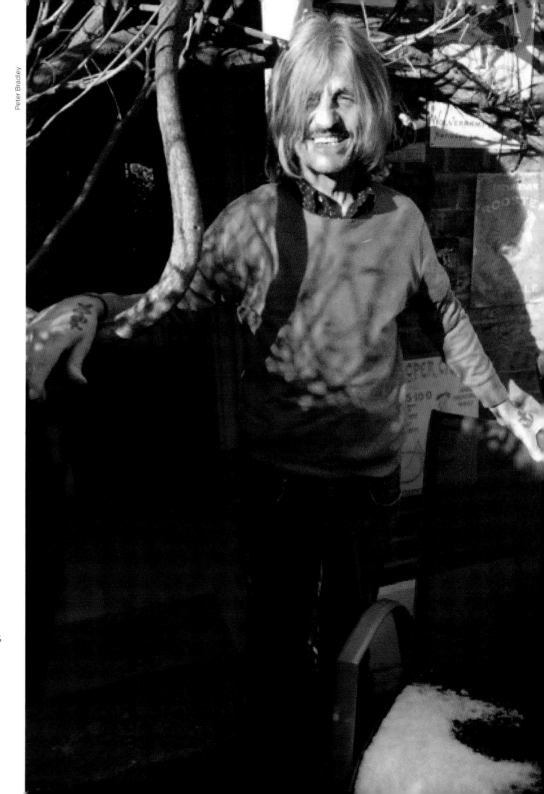

Peter Bradley

Tommy Hanchen
Two Bag Tommy

I'll get to the title a little later. You can keep guessing if you like, but I'd bet you'd not figure it out. For 30 years, come rain or shine, I've been an ardent lover of the Blue. Through all my ups and downs and still going strong. Well just about for now. Come next week, I'm having major surgery to remove yet another cancer that has been part of my life for the past ten years.

This short piece about my love of cold water swimming is not about my health struggles. Yet the Blue continues to

be a major part of my recovery and amazing health, in spite of it all. When I've been in hospital, I dream about swimming again and I'm convinced it drives my motivation to be discharged as soon as I can. Sometimes against the wishes of the doctors, but I'll be back in the water as soon as I can walk.

I remember listening to a committed cold water swimming doctor explain how there's little hard evidence of how cold water swimming is good for your health. However, there's no doubt that he and his fellow swimmers all feel tremendously good after their swims. To which the interviewer responds without missing a beat, 'but if you were hit over the head with a hammer and then that stopped, wouldn't you also feel tremendously good?'

Well there is that, I suppose. Like the good doctor said, I don't know about the evidence of the benefits. I do know that me and my fellow swimmers are guaranteed to also feel tremendously good every time without fail. This is not some form of perverted masochism, it's the best high of the day. Being an old git now, I get the old git pass and swim for free. How good is that?

It amuses me how us early birds gather at break of day mostly in silence and half asleep, as if guided by some invisible, mysterious force.

Just watch how this changes post-swim. As though we have all been given a large dose of amphetamine, everyone is talking and laughing that high-energy speedy talk. Magic; if I could bottle this effect, I would. Now many years ago, if you visited the Blue when the sun was high in the sky you entered a community of many villages. Settled around the pool with their territorial boundaries clearly marked. There you'd find the single mums, the families, the brothers and sisters and Rastas, gay boys and girls, with the odds and ends where ever they can. A wonderful and peaceful example of diversity, you might say. On one such day, I wish I had recorded the following dialogue which caught the attention of the whole community, who laughed and heckled as one. From the days when there was a tannoy in reception :
"Winston, there's a pizza been delivered for you in reception."
(remember it's a blistering hot day)
10 minutes later and impatiently
"Winston, your pizza is getting cold!"
Finally and 10 minutes later still
"Winston, if you don't come now, I'll eat the damn thing!" Only in Brixton-on-sea. Back to the title. My cancer left me with a colostomy bag and after next week I'll have a bag for my urine too. All my plumbing on the outside, hence: Two Bag Tommy.

In all these years I've been swimming freely and entirely comfortable with showering and changing. Never a funny look or whispered conversation.

I can't tell you enough how good that feels to be accepted like that.
So here I am coming to the end of this piece with my heartfelt thanks. To all the people, staff and committees that keep this wonderful place going. To all my fellow nutters, well we have to be a little nuts, who rise at the crack of dawn for their daily fix.

Our father, Tom Hanchen, sadly passed away on 1 November 2020 at 67 years of age—although we are happy to report that dad's urostomy and the loss of the use of one leg did not keep him away from the water! Two Bag Tommy continued to love swimming at Brockwell Park Lido and the joy it would give him was deeply inspiring and infectious!
Chloë and Yolande Hanchen

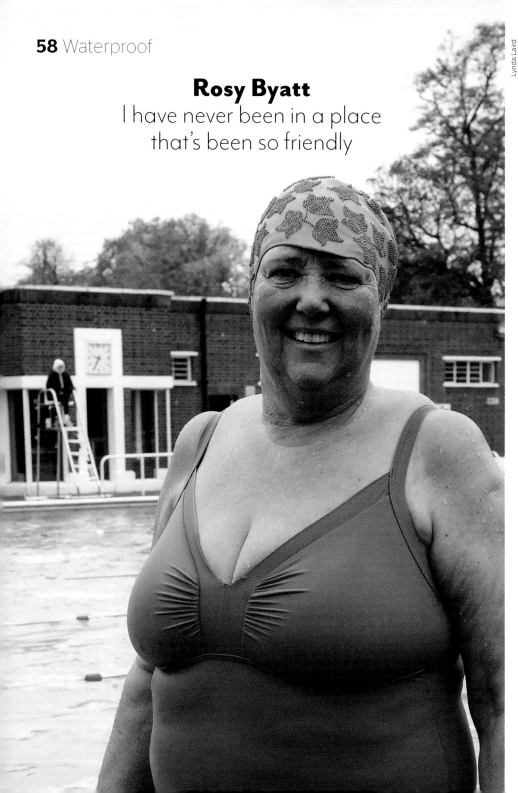

Lynda Laird

Rosy Byatt
I have never been in a place that's been so friendly

My Lido experience begins with a bike ride from home through two beautiful parks: Dulwich and Brockwell. All year round, I notice the seasons changing, the trees, the sky, the air. I love the whole season thing, I love them all. Each day's different, the light's different, the sky darkening or lightening. The journey is a major part of coming here. Even if it's grey, it doesn't matter, it's still atmospheric. It's a sort of ritual, cycling here.

Then you come into the changing room and it's full of friendly people. You see people you know and take part in the friendly chatter and banter. You hear the men next door laughing in their changing room.

I love the turquoise colour of the pool, the quality of the water and the colour of the light. Even if it's cloudy, it's just a different colour. Then there's the patterns the sun makes on the bottom of the pool. Each day it's a different sensation.

Swimming for me is a meditative experience. Because it's quite a long pool, it's a sort of meditation for me and, I think, for lots of people. I am so busy in the rest of my life with work and family, but swimming is something I do just for myself. That's really important.

In winter, the sun is very low and the light very different. I love the big expanse of the sky here, that 360 degree view you get. And I love the trees around the Lido and I always look at them. In winter, they're little

bare sticks and overnight, it seems, they're suddenly quite bushy. It's not gradual, but immediate.

Then there is the friendliness. I have never been in a place that's been so friendly. I have made a lot of friends here: you can never have enough friends, in my opinion.

When I've finished swimming, I feel, I've had my time for myself. It sets the day up in a different way. I try not to book any patient in before 11am.

I come as often as I can, four days a week or so. I used to feel guilty if I couldn't come every day, now I feel it's good to come when I can make it and I don't feel guilty at all, just enjoy it when I'm here.

This is my second winter swimming through the whole winter. A couple of times before, I stopped when I got to November or December. Last year, when I'd swum through the whole winter for the first time, I was pleased I had done it. Once you carry on, it's fine; it's when you stop that it's difficult.
I enjoy the cold water and the feeling of it on my skin. It's exhilarating and I miss it when I can't make it. I find it addictive. And on cold days, you know you can have a hot shower afterwards—and then on to breakfast in the Lido Café, or outside on warmer days.
I would find it very hard to move away from the Lido. It's such a draw. You couldn't recreate it elsewhere, it's a mixture of things

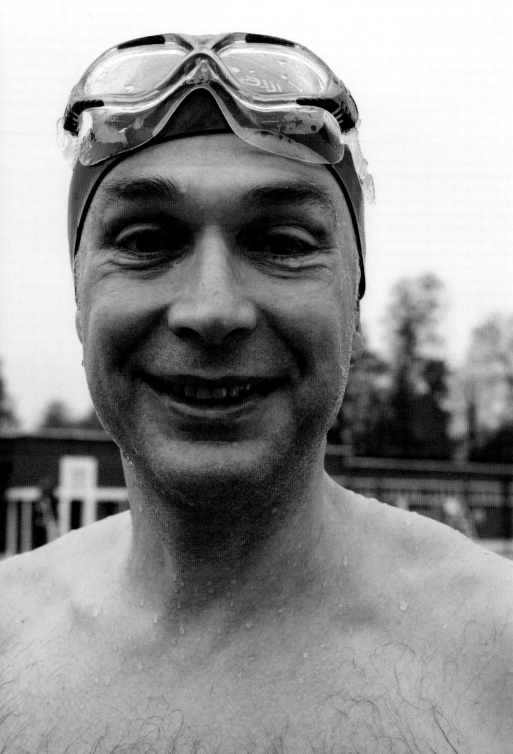

Lynda Laird

Stephen Trowell
Do not mistake the Lido in Winter for the Summer water that laughs and plays

Do not mistake the Lido in Winter for the Summer water that laughs and plays

Why get into that cold, cold water? It is easy to answer on a sunny Winter's day when the water is made of diamonds and the only surprise is that all of South London is not diving in for some of the riches.

It is easy to answer from the café, with a coffee in hand, bundled against the cold, when the swim is over and one feels good and something, at least, has been achieved.

But on the cloudy, wine-dark days when the rain is about to fall, when there is old grit on the paving stones from last week's frost, and the grey water is massed against you, why, why then get into that cold, cold water? Do not doubt: the water will take your breath; the cold will first burn you and then freeze you—your fingers and toes, your legs and arms; and, though only you will know, as your head goes under, your brain will scream.

When you first start to swim, the water does not let you through. You might thrash your arms against the cold, but you will be held like a bird flying against the wind. Respect must be paid. Do not mistake the Lido in Winter for the Summer water that laughs and plays and trickles from your skin. The Winter twin demands your body whole, again and again, before she will yield to you. Then, after a hard-fought length, the water starts to let you through. You pull on it, thick in your hands, and it pushes you faster and faster. The dark day does not matter, the grey rain is unnoticed, because all there is, is the cold water and you.

Do not try and stay in the joy of that moment too long because every part of it is paid for with your heat, and if you stay too long, too much will be taken.

So take those minutes in the cold, cold water between home and work, and live outside your normal day.

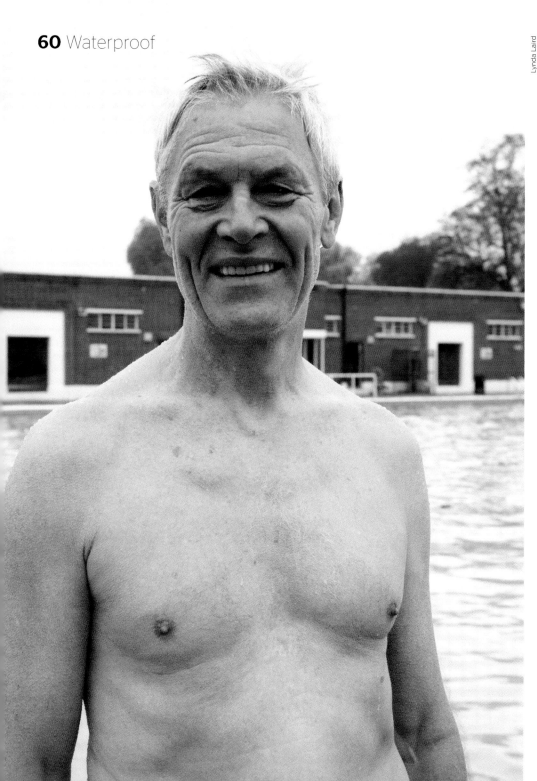

Lynda Laird

Michael Wynn
Only the body and the water. All blue and cold

It's a cold grey November morning. Not quite frosty, but it's been a cold deep night. A rising mist in the park as I tiptoe into the Lido. My pulse rises imperceptibly as I gaze over that blue oblong of cold water. Just a frisson of anticipation. I casually inspect the water temperature out of sheer habit. Has it gone down? Have we reached the magic below fifty yet? The Bec (Tooting Bec) and the Serps (Serpentine) are already telling the world they're down at at 48. No worries. Eleven centigrade can't harm anyone!

Leave the woolly hat behind and I begin the long walk from the changing room to the Deep End. Good morning to our faithful lifeguards. Drape same towel on same rail. Brave the cold shower. Adjust reality. Abandon last sense of comfort—the flipflops at pool end. Ready stop watch. And now 'Die Stunde ist gekommen' (the hour has come). One last stare at the far end. Deep breath. In head first. Feel the tingle. Cold fire. Breathe. Deep. Control the lungs. Keep the head low. Stare at the myriad bubbles rising.

Head up to snatch more breath. More bubbles rising. Look up. The far end closer now. Nearly there. Touch cold concrete. Kick off. Check the watch. A good first fifty always warms you up! Now settle into lazy breast stroke and enjoy the swim. Glance around. Four or five others immersed in water. Each to own thoughts. Do I think when I'm in the pool? Not a lot. It's the senses. Now I'm alive. The old thoughts don't leave me. But now they're dressed in a different garb. It's the water pressing on my skin. It's the cold creeping in. Let it settle in deep. I'm in my body now and my body is afire. The limbs are loose. The muscles are plasticine. The skin is taut. Knots of flesh in the blue cold deep of the Lido. I look up. The comfort of the slow ticking clock a reminder of a time-bound world that I left only moments ago. This new world is a cold, fluid, expanding and contracting

universe. My lungs in tune with the deep. My slippery self wrapped in cold cocoon. Equipoised between water and air surface. Light refracting. Nostrils blowing bubbles. Cheek bones like ice creams.

Five lengths. The fluid blue oblong. The swimmer. The air above. The brick surround. The clock. Tree branches in cold Arctic currents. The park. The morning dogs out sniffing. The red buses beyond.

Six lengths. The oblong. The cold swimmers. The goggles and hats. Air in the lungs. The beyond.

Seven lengths. The oblong beneath. The long smooth convex beneath. All in blue. Gasping. Washed bodies. Wet souls. Breath diminished. Breath expanded. Heads bobbing.

Eight. Is it cold enough? When does the body freeze? When is time to stop? Nine. Push off. Only the body and the water. All blue and cold.
Ten. Enough. Now touch in. Check the watch. Dive down and touch below. Up. Rest. Pull up. Out. Watch and steady. Readjust to surface pressure. Cold shower.

Now the stone flags and a certain course to the little warm hut. Inside the glow of warm flesh. Animated box with a hundred voices. Babbling. 20, 30, 2ks. Below fifty. Siberia. Ice holes. No end of chatter. Some shiver. Some laugh. Some immersed in feeling the thaw. Bodies warming. Water splashing from the wooden spoon. Scent of pine. Each of us just starting a day. In our own way.

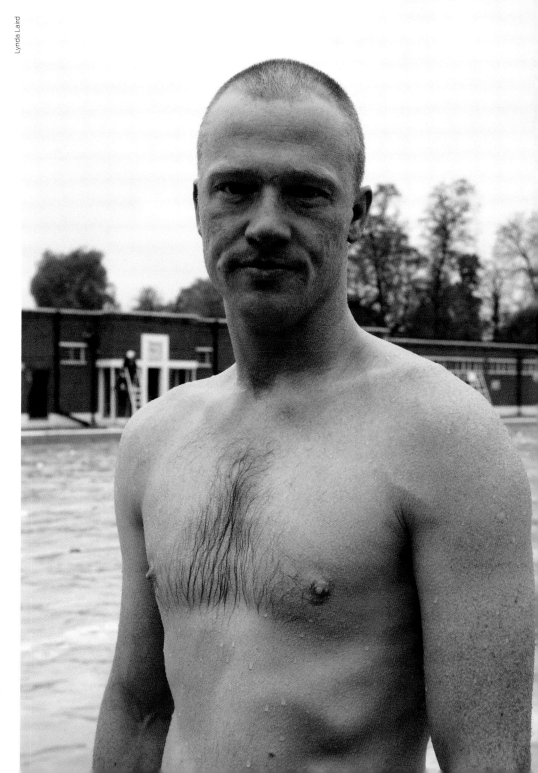

Lynda Laird

Ian Thel
Was it cold? Describe ...

I can't claim to know the full experience of winter swimming. Till now, I've pushed only as far as the autumn with its crisp, gleaming mornings. So this account is liable to privilege the romantic over the plain painful. Others will know more about that. But I've long known something of the impulse to take to frigid water.

As a teenager holidaying in the Scottish Islands, I would blithely brave the Firth of Clyde, sheltered by the mass of Arran and the Hebrides behind me, and by the Holy Isle filling the better part of the bay in front. At these latitudes, summer is fleeting, so although in June the water wouldn't reach much over 11 or 12 degrees,

the opportunity to get wet on the occasional sunnier day was never lost. Invariably the first to wade in, I remember calling to timid friends and relatives on shore: 'it's OK, you won't feel the cold once you're numb!'

Though sure to encourage numbness, swimming in the cold water of Brockwell seems to me more than a simple case of anaesthesia. Unlike the ecstatic release of spontaneous immersion in wilder spots, there is a more deliberate catharsis in its enforced and repetitive insistence not only on letting go enough to take the plunge, but on holding on once in. This persistence achieves a worldly kind of isolation, one that transcends the more prosaic experience of the indoor pool. Swimming here is—as it was for Burt Lancaster's amnesiac patriarch in the 1968 movie, *The Swimmer*—a matter of forgetting and coming to remembrance all at the same time. Perhaps it's just the relative emptiness here at the Lido—and I've more than once had the luxury of this whole expanse to myself—that encourages this. It's also surely the openness to the sky, making for a near absence of reflected sound. It's also the unusual clarity of the water, at least once the holidays are done, and the play of cool, autumn sunlight as it refracts through the chop into a web on the floor. Most important, though, is the sudden compression the body experiences as it enters the water: the tightening of the chest; the necessity to push all air from the lungs; the acute awareness of the skin, now stinging, as a kind of limit. It's this that ultimately pushes all considerations inward.

This acute disruption has for me the effect of expelling all thoughts, all that interior monologue. It's a lurch from a basic mental state of distraction, to a bodily concentration on the crucial matters of stroke, breath, keeping the eyes to the surface, staying long, relaxing. Here, if you can hold on, not only can the outside world be lost, but the act of swimming itself can become transparent too. Here, suspended in light, with full goggle vision, tiny bubbles tracing my fingertips as they stretch a path out front, I have sometimes come close to what I know from dreams to be the sensation of flying: innate responsiveness; a fantasy conveyed by water, borne out by a struggling body, striving to reach that moment—rare as Scottish sun—where its movements somehow coalesce in an impression of effortlessness. In moments such as these, the mind can be encouraged to transpose this particular body of water to a host

of others swum in the past: torrid meltwater in the French Alps; shocking glacial pools in Iceland; silt-infused zones of the Channel and the North Sea; vegetal upper reaches of the Thames; brackish pools discovered between Highland waterfalls; semi-saline lochs. Most memorably, for me, though, these moments transplant precious, crystalline swims over the shell-sands of Barra, Islay, Tiree: Brockwell Lido, at its best, is my own shivering slab of cold, Hebridean Atlantic.

Needless to say, all this lasts the shortest of whiles. Soon, and likely sooner as the days draw in and the temperature drops, the cold that gave brief permission to these reveries barges them out again, returning me to my body. At 10 degrees, the muscles tire quickly, the breath becomes ragged, and the water that seemed so encouraging before

becomes harder, heavier, wholly non-compliant. Extremities begin to squeal in complaint and lips—even teeth—register pain.

Yet these are not the feelings I take away after a swim here. As the blood begins to work back outwards from the centre, and I carry this inner warmth into the day, I find whatever mental knots and clumps came with me have been quietly disassembled and re-ordered behind my back. In this way, the masochistic desire to persist in a situation that ought to trigger flight allows me to remain grounded as I carry on with whatever else might occupy me, outside of this transformative place.

Mike Richardson
An hour of holiday a day

If I swam every day that would be 365 hours.
45 eight-hour days. 2 months, 9 working weeks, a holiday ...

With pre-holiday anticipation I've been swimming whilst I slept.
Glinting rays on the Art Deco windows slightly blind the eye.
The building where long summers are spent and happy memories kept.
It's cheap, deep and laden with 1930s swimming zest.

Laughter swims already from the Ladies' changing away.
All bodies are beautiful here, all shapes and lines and creases.
Everything goes, no judgements are made when we're on display.
This is for each and every one of us an hour of holiday.

Swoon into the water, bird of prey.
Soothing the pains throughout the vertebrae.
The healing of cold softens our decay.
To a brighter perspective, this is the gateway.

The water has its merits in all of the different seasons.
Winter sometimes makes you question,
But the dense cold pool returns you to your reason.
More cold means more tea, jumpers, sauna and camaraderie.

In Spring, green returns to trees, sensation to the fingers.
A hesitant entry rewards, and the grind in your mind dwindles.
From the sauna seeing stars while the fresh morning light lingers.
The energy from the pool is yours to keep and tomorrow rekindle.

Summer brings the rest of town for their various holidays.
Molecules racing the water's at its lightest, shorts,
Shouts, screams, jumps, more bodies on display.
It's not long before we long for Autumn and its less busy days.

This is the most exciting time of year.
The water gradually thickens bottom up.
The first leaves in the pool, the first chill in the air.
The knowledge that our friends alone will soon be here.

Alone but together we will keep our holiday.
As seasons change and temperatures fluctuate.
So does sauna, chat, wetsuits and trips to the café.
As we jubilantly enact this impossible ballet.

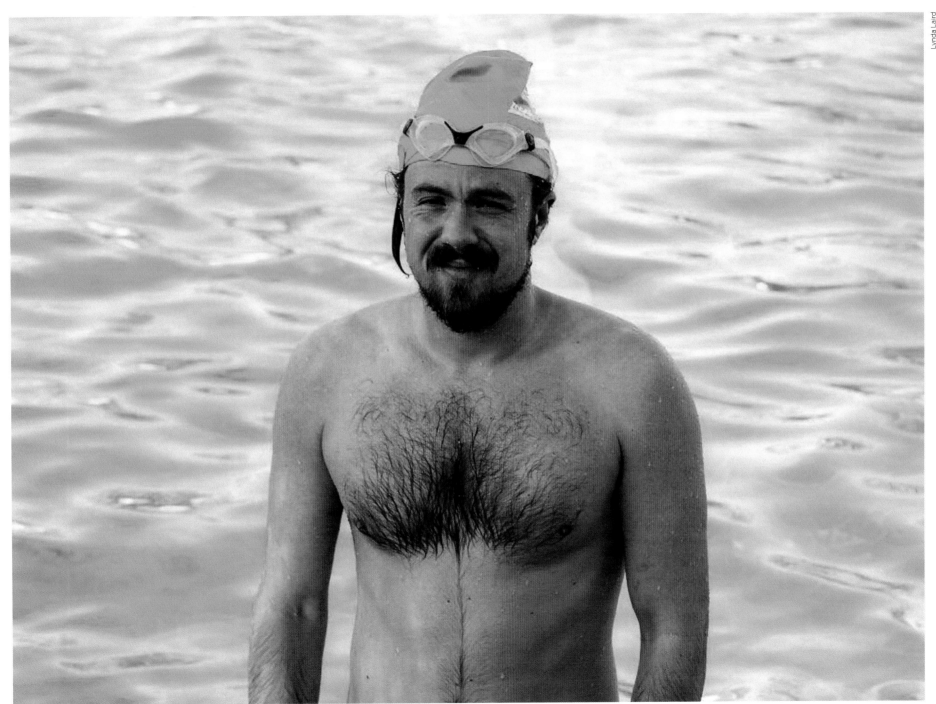

Mark Woodhead (right)
Impluvium—poem and illustration

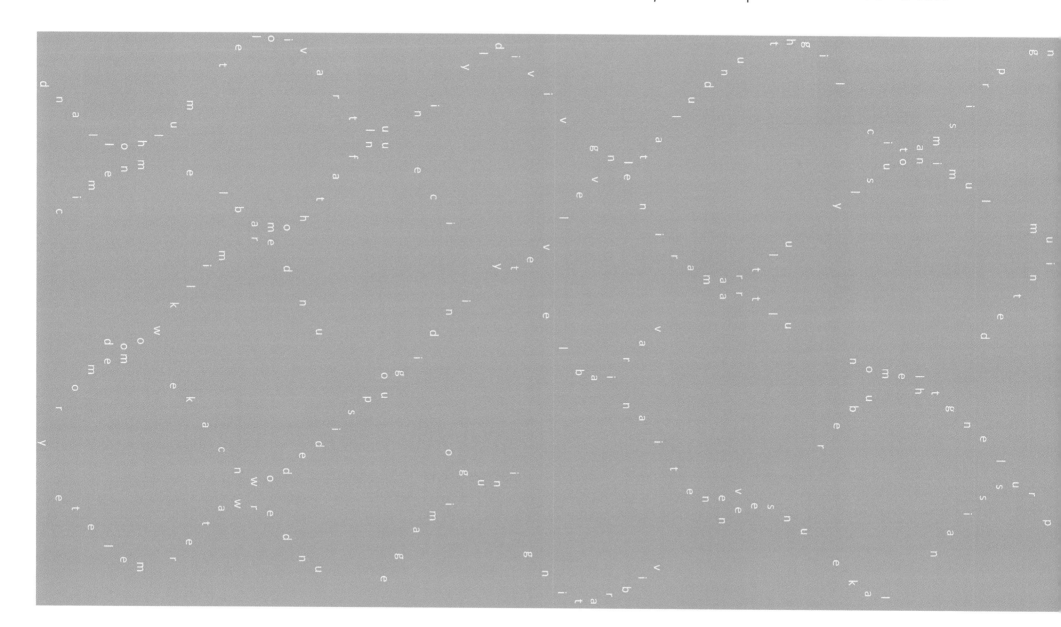

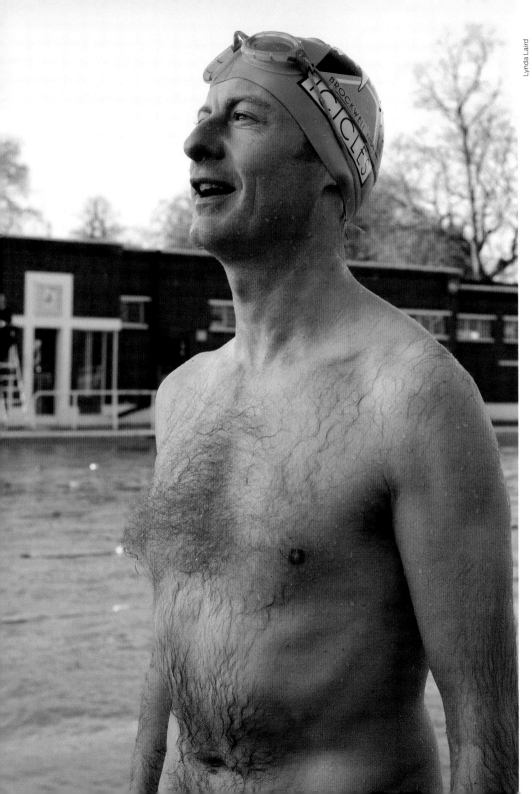

Lynda Laird

Chapter 4

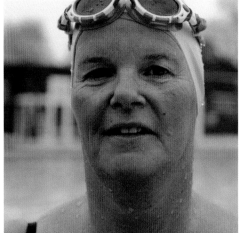

Marc Woodhead 66
impluvium
Lido Mike and Lido Sarah 68
We were both hooked on cold water and open water swimming
John Finlay 70
Truants
Mark Frost 72
By the third length, without fail I am in heaven
Jason Homewood 74
From the lifeguard chair
Sebastian Hepher 75
Why do you swim in the Lido in winter?
Chris Roberts 76
Not just the pool

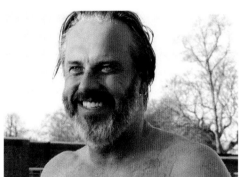

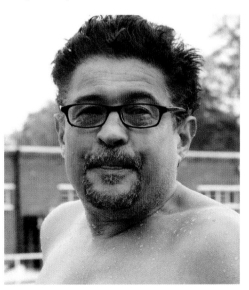

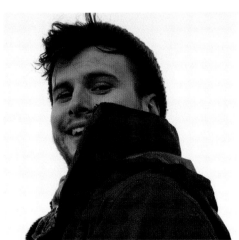

'Lido Mike' and 'Lido Sarah' Johnstone
We were both hooked on cold water and open water swimming

Cool swims
Tingle pain biting fresh
Thrill happy cool lap
smooth floaty icey bite
Choppy sunlight
waves laugh
Bright blue flicker patterns
leaves hang
Slow motion air wind
breeze chill
Surge boost alive
Space open breathe sky
Length happy dancing
Sparkle rhythm
Beat heart ease relax
soften time melt.
Lido Mike

Cold water swimming
You must be crazy,
they say!
But, minus the chill, thrill,
time standing still,
Who knows how crazy
I'd be?
Lido Sarah

Swimming lifeline
Swimming is not just great
for your mind and body,
it's an essential life skill that
gives you the ability and
confidence to enjoy so
many other water-based
activities. It has provided
us with great experiences,
challenges and fun. We
have found swimming,
particularly in cold water,
to be the perfect antidote
to the stress and strain of
inner city life.
We grew up together and
in the late 1960s both
learnt to swim in Ladywell
indoor 33-metre pool. You
had to be quite brave to
survive the freezing cold
changing rooms and the
power-crazed attendants,
who would shout at you
if you forgot your locker
number. In the 1970s and

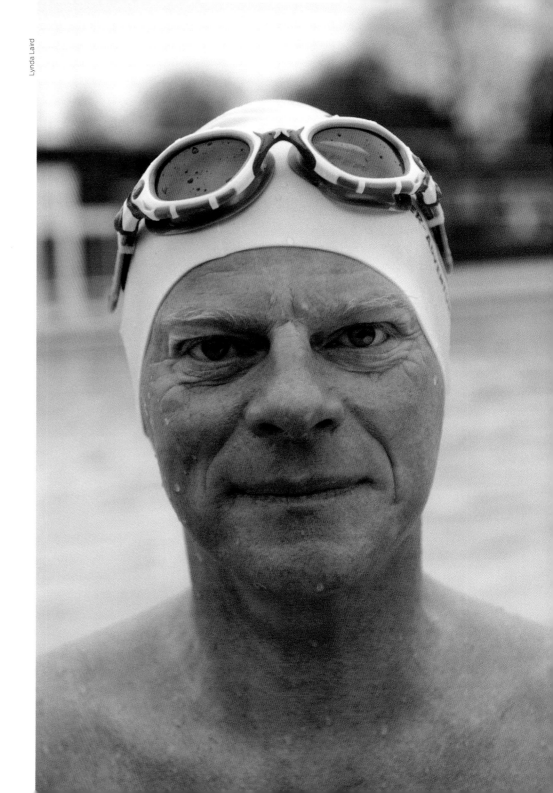

Lynda Laird

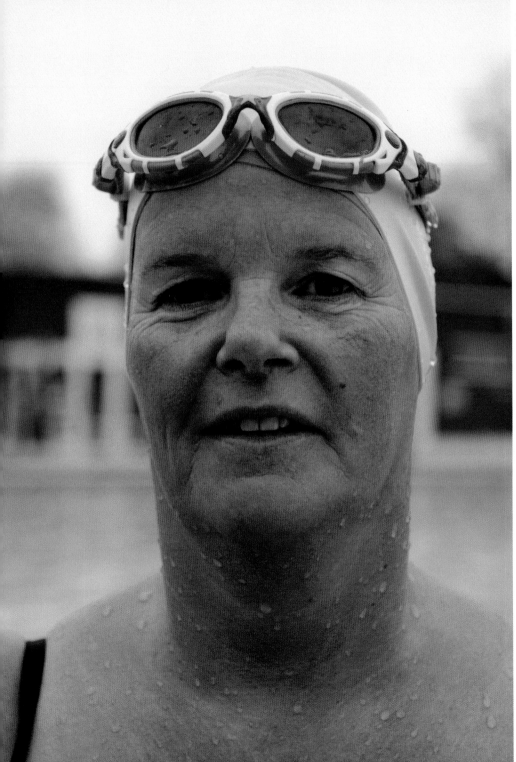

Lynda Laird

early 1980s, we swam in various unheated Lidos, such as Charlton, Peckham, and Southwark Park before they sadly closed. Eltham Park, built in 1924, was one of our favourites; set in a well-kept park, it had a sun deck and café and we would spend all day there whenever we could. Minehead Lido (165 ft x 60 ft and 15 ft deep) in Somerset was a holiday destination, with a huge 33 ft diving platform. Opened in 1936, it was right on the sea front and apparently filled every day with 50 000 gallons of filtered sea water per hour!

As young adults, we both got hooked on cold water and open water swimming: wherever we went, whatever the water temperature, we had to swim in seas, lakes, rivers and lidos (not always popular once we had

children, who sometimes complained that all we ever did was swim!).

In the late 1980s, we discovered Tooting Lido and spent many summers and winters relaxing and swimming there.

Now our spring and summers are happily spent poolside at wonderful Brockwell Lido, working together as Streamline Swims, enjoying teaching and coaching swimmers of all ages and abilities and fitting in a few lengths and open water challenges when we can.

Once autumn and winter come, it's lovely to have more time to swim, chat and celebrate with others what we all love about Brockwell lido and the magic of cold water swimming.

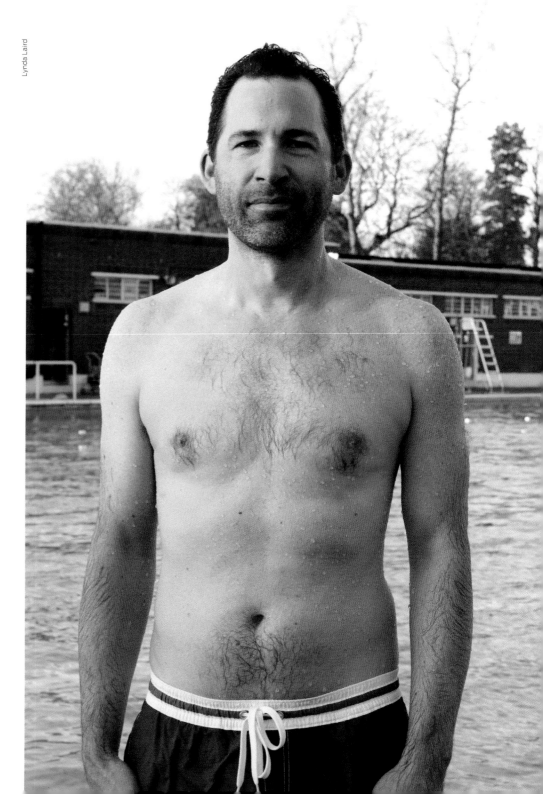

Lynda Laird

John Finlay
Truants

I knew someone once who took part in one of those extreme charity events. You know, the ones where you're generally required to push yourself to traumatising levels of physical exertion, but which at the same time have the capacity to make your distant, sedentary audience just a little jealous of the once-in-a-lifetime experience you're having.

His challenge was an unassisted group trek to the North Pole, or somewhere in that direction, and one compulsory element of trip preparation was the cold water test. In just swimming costumes, they had to jump into arctic water through a paddling-pool-sized hole in some thick ice. Ideally they then had to get themselves out again

too—I don't think they were allowed to go if they couldn't ... It seemed an impressive, almost aspirational act to be able to achieve, yet something you would clearly always avoid if given the choice.

Apart from this and seeing the Christmas Serpentine swimmers in the papers each year, my knowledge of proper cold water swimming was very limited until I started my working life next to the Lido. Although I can swim, I'm certainly not a swimmer and not someone that often takes exercise at all just for the sake of it. From memory, I may not have swum once in the Lido during the first summer I worked here, warm as it was. However, I gradually became aware of the people that just didn't stop swimming, once it began to get cold and miserable outside. I struggled to see the appeal.

This is not to say that there were too many of them. Lack of full winter opening just a few years ago meant many eventually had to look elsewhere for their off-season dips. Once this changed, a sprinkling of people would still swim in the limited times the pool was open, but the need for most to get to work, and simply get warm again, didn't make for too much hanging around and chatting afterwards. By the time habit-forming daily winter swims were possible, the same shivering faces began to appear at the terrace door more and more often. As the weeks and months went by, that number, each wearing about four coats and struggling to get their words out, eventually became conspicuous. As 'gourmet' and above the coffee mainstream as we aspire to be, our modestly sized hot drinks were struggling to win the warming challenge they faced, and so we began to offer them at half-price to those who'd braved the pool once it dipped below 10 degrees.

Having spent so long in witness to their routine of daily physical epiphany, there would always be a day when I would have to try it myself. After probably two and a half years of nagging (I'm thinking of you, Peretz ...), I finally showed up one cloudy November morning to surprise the main group. Even at the best of times, I can't swim more than a length of the Lido without stopping, so I didn't have high targets set for myself, but the effects of water colder than I'd ever been in before were still a surprise. I bit the bullet and waded in confidently, but despite an unexpected initial optimism once I started, the inevitable sensation of slowing-motion took hold soon after about half-way.

I think I can recognise the potential for exhilaration from the surreal effects of the cold numbing your body. The downside is that, if you aren't used to that feeling, your body soon stops doing what you ask of it and you realise that you're likely to sink unless you get out pretty quickly. I just about made it to the steps at the end of that first length, but getting up them never quite felt guaranteed. The whole

escapade was quite a revelation, but be very sure that 6°C water will get the better of you sooner than you think. Despite having only repeated the experience once more since then (even colder, even more terrifying), the impression you get of others enjoying their ritual is one of their overriding happiness in doing so. Almost no-one forces anyone to swim in cold water, with the rarest of exceptions, and yet the reward for those that do seems so comfortably to outweigh the discomfort that they come back for more, time and time again.

Not many a morning goes by in the Café where people don't ask, 'is the pool heated?' and if it's not the height of summer, they'll look at you in rarely-veiled shock when you tell them it's not. 'But there are people swimming, without wetsuits?' they say, and we'll reply with something along the lines of 'yes, but it's still a bit warm for the crazy ones that come all year round'. The 'Icicles' will forgive me, I think, for questioning their sanity—I'm pretty confident it's a badge of honour they proudly wear on their many layers of swimming hats. There is a palpable

sense of disappointment each year if there isn't at least some snow on the coldest days.

Not just here, but for probably a great majority of cold-swimmers, the role of cake in the recovery process is pretty indisputable. The penchant for competitive home-baking among our adopted group can therefore be something of a silent battlefront. As you'd imagine, we're hard at work selling our own wares to the rest of our visitors each day, so bribery to overlook crumb-strewn surroundings is not unheard of. However, their looks of nervous guilt when they think they've pushed things a bit far makes too stern a reaction difficult.

More often than not, at gone 10 in the morning a few survivors will still be sat at our big table by the bar. We quietly wonder if in fact they do still have jobs to go to? It seems that truancy when you have something wild to do is not something that's left behind after childhood.

Lynda Laird

Mark Frost
By the third length, without fail I am in heaven

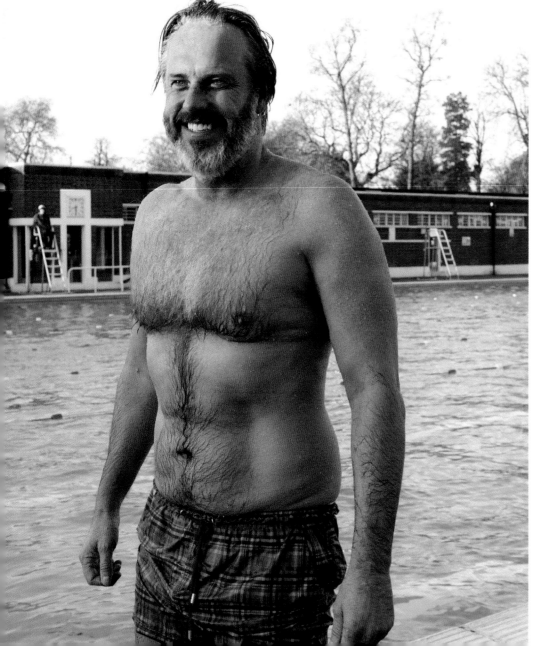

I am a winter Brockwell virgin. Today was my first sub-10 degrees plunge ... there have been many such firsts in the preceding months, but with a heavy autumn frost forecast for this evening I am entering uncharted territory and I am excited.

I have caught the bug ...

On awakening, my body is up and out the door before the mind has had a chance to argue ...

The cold water takes hold of you ... gets in your bones ... becomes a craving ... an obsession. How low can you go?

My neighbour looks at me like I am mad as, the night before, she emerges wrapped up and comments on the chill, and I tell her excitedly 'the pool will be cold in the morning'. That is part of the thrill ... the secret pleasure ... misunderstood by the uninitiated. On the days when I haven't been able to get my fix, I am sluggish, irritable and discontent.
Travelling out of town these days necessitates checking in with the other 'Icicles' to get insider tips on wild swimming spots, or trawling the internet in search of watering holes in which to immerse oneself. Sometimes, outings away from the Lido are taken with my fellow cold water adherents and become a great source of joy. These

may involve housewarmings (at a self-built coastal dwelling of an ex-Icicle, whose pool has become the ocean on her doorstep), or a show, or a gallery, but always a swim or two is prioritised in the schedule. This ragtag bunch of cold water disciples, the 'Icicles', has become as much a source of joy as the chilly lido swim itself.

I first encountered this group in April around the poolside picnic table adjacent to the café. I had always admired the architecture of Brockwell Lido, was a big fan of the park and had used the gym sporadically and the pool a handful of times, along with the summer throng, but hadn't fully appreciated its charms. A friend, Steffan, had just completed his first winter and spoke of this singular lido experience with unbridled fervour and a fanatical look in his eye. He encouraged me to give it a go and so, at the beginning of April, I started dipping on a daily basis. The 13 or 14 degrees of the early spring water seemed reasonable enough. I didn't quite see what all the fuss was about. I managed a handful of lengths, alternating an ungainly crawl with a tired breaststroke and then sheepishly joined my friend at the picnic table in among the 'Icicles'. This disparate group all shared my friend's fervour and his fanatical gleam. They talked in a language I didn't wholly understand while eating their pre-prepared breakfasts from various containers, the merits of which were up for analysis along with the water conditions, the quality of the light, the state of play in the organisation of the Lido and other pressing local matters. There was much excitement this year after the installation of an outdoor sauna, shaped like a gypsy caravan, which sat next to the pool, and there were various debates on how best to enjoy the swim/sauna combination or 'double-dip' that it provided (swim–sauna–second dip in the pool).

I didn't quite know as yet what all the fuss was about, but I secretly wanted to belong ... to be accepted. Some mornings, home-made cakes or cookies or banana bread were on offer and shared out among the gathering. There was an openness, an ease and a welcoming generosity around the bench that was infectious. As the summer hordes arrived and the water became cloudy with sunscreen, world affairs would occasionally impinge on the badinage of the picnic bench. For a while, Brexit rocked the bench and gave a rare gravitas to proceedings ... but breakfast was never too serious for too long. Matters inevitably returned to the rhythms of the Lido ... who had the best stroke, the state of the café porridge, the algae on the floor of the pool and other pressing concerns ... always with wit, warmth and laughter

... after all, this was a place one came to escape the pressures of the world outside. That said, individual problems could be shared and the group would instantly rally round. I was sharing chocolate cake at the bench one morning when I received a call from my sister in Australia to say that her husband, Peter, had passed away in the night; I was immediately moved by the simple generosity of this bunch of relative strangers. I realised that this 'therapy' bench was as much a part of the Lido experience as the swim itself.

I came to appreciate the various characters who worked at the Lido, or in the café and the numerous invigorated post-swim faces from a host of regulars, some of whom I recognised from other walks and my decade of living in the neighbouring area. I shared daily observations on the latest swim while warming up in the sauna. I met Casey, who had saved the Lido years earlier, and heard his tales of wilder times with late night parties, naked swims and a more relaxed organisation.

I felt childish glee when I first started swimming only crawl, and again a few weeks later when I swam my first kilometre. We made excursions to Parliament Hill Lido for magical moonlit swims in September. I received helpful emails detailing potential

outdoor swims while I was working away and unable to join my Brockwell breakfast club. One trip with a pair of 'Icicles' to see Steffan in a play in Chichester involved us sharing a yurt, much hilarity and an unforgettable misty morning swim in Bosham Harbour. Indeed, the mornings have become a totally new experience, involving an appreciation of the movements of the seasons and the ever-changing early luminescence, that would otherwise go unnoticed. Now that the temperature is dropping, sometimes suddenly a couple of degrees in as many days, the first length is a challenge and inevitably involves having to have a word with myself as I catch my breath at the far end and face the hazy morning sun. By the third length, without fail I am in heaven, thrown back into the moment ... and the breath ... and the stroke.

I have grown to love the idiosyncrasies of the members of the 'Icicle' family, chuckling at Peter's daily naked phoned order to the café from the changing room, so that once clad his porridge awaits (no pre-prepared tupperware fayre for him), or Katie's origami creations or Liz's inspirational ideas for illicit swimming adventure. Different hours bring a slightly different crowd, no less eager or engaging and gradually most of the faces become familiar. Some leave for a while, taken

away by work, but always return with gratitude, ready to worship in the waters again. It has already been a transcendent experience and new activities have resulted from my simple saying yes to the swim some seven or so months ago. We have been Northern soul dancing, taken part in Lido Café barista Andrea's gong baths and meditations and other socials, but in the end it is all about the swim.

I bought my winter ticket today and while I sat at breakfast (indoors in the café in November) David (Grafton) whispered to me, 'can I interest you in a new swimming cap?'

This is it ... the 'Icicle' badge of honour, this year in a fetching pink, had hitherto been talked about in hushed tones ... all very secretive ... supply uncertain and anticipation high.
Suddenly, simple as that, there it is ... £6.50 and I have one ...
I'm in the club ...
I belong ...
The Lido and its inhabitants have won my heart. The simple act of saying yes to a bracing morning swim seven and a bit months ago has opened up a whole new world.
There is no turning back.
Brockwell Lido provides a complete attitude adjuster and I love it.

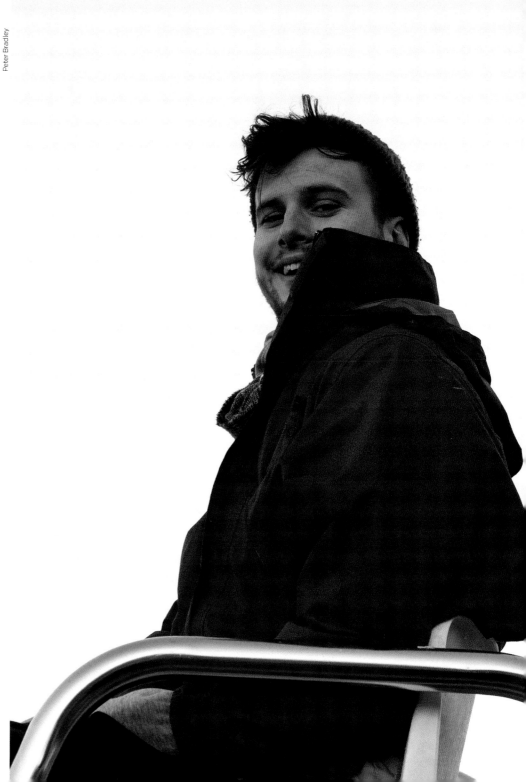

Peter Bradley

Jason Homewood
From the lifeguard chair

I have been a lifeguard on and off for around 6 years, I have worked in a variety of centres and come in contact with an awful lot of the people. Out of all them, Brockwell Lido is a brand new experience! Whether that's the outdoors and current 8 degrees pool temperature I don't know, but there is definitely something different about this pool. In all honesty, I think it's the people! There's got to be something in that water that makes everyone so happy—it's a pleasure to be around people who actually say good morning and as a lifeguard treat you like you're human. During the winter periods, I enjoy watching people struggle and fight with the absurdly cold water. I feel like I'm going through it with them as the wind batters my face on the lifeguard chair. And at the back of my mind I'm constantly thinking, 'please don't drown!'. During summer, the pool becomes alive ... there's people everywhere and my job becomes a lot harder. But working outside with the sun beating down, it's pretty great— much better than an indoor pool that feels like you're in a greenhouse! I'm not going to be at Brockwell for much longer, but I'd like to say thank you to the swimmers in the morning who give us a smile, start a conversation and are crazy enough to be in that water at its temperature: you make the early mornings a bit more bearable.
Jason Homewood
(The lifeguard always in a hat)

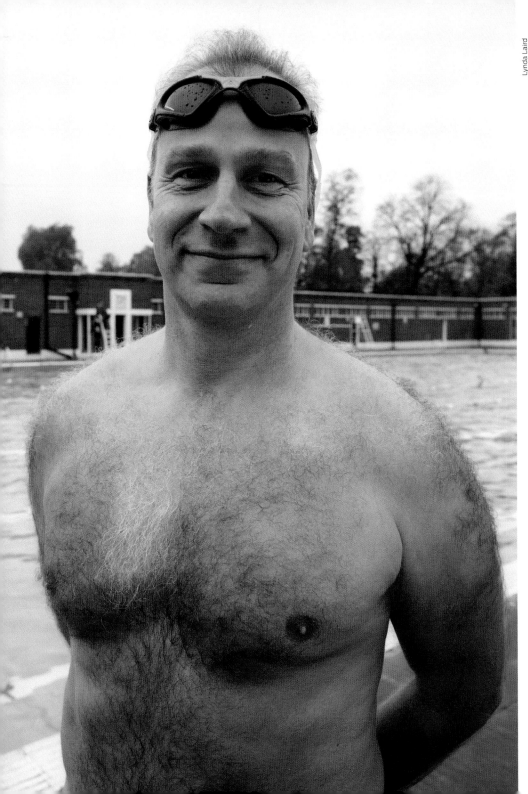

Lynda Laird

Sebastian Hepher
Why do you swim in the Lido in winter?

Why do you swim in the Lido in winter? Perhaps it is because, as the cold water closes over one's body and the sounds of the great city awakening are swallowed, one has a complete sense of release. There is a theory that plunging into water of 7 degrees and below so shocks the body that all of its energies are focused on survival. Is it that which allows the mind to forget all that has happened, or that which lies ahead, and to focus for a precious few minutes each day on the present, without interference or disturbance?

Gradually, the body adjusts to the temperature and the initial, brutal pain is replaced by a numb acceptance. The beauty of the Lido then becomes apparent. The trees, with branches as bare as those of the swimmers, stand sentinel to the walled haven below. Those swimmers, sporting their colourful and seasonal hats, share a common bond; an understanding of and mutual respect for all that it means to be one of the few who brave the wintery waters. The café, with the warm aroma of pastries and coffee, offers a tantalising yet premature sanctuary as the lengths mount up. The decking, which in summer is a mass of seasonal guests, lies bare and clear, flanked by the wisteria-clad walls. The open sky forms a roof of endless design and pattern which on a crisp, sunny day is enough to raise even the lowest of spirits.

Why do I swim in the Lido in winter?

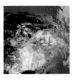

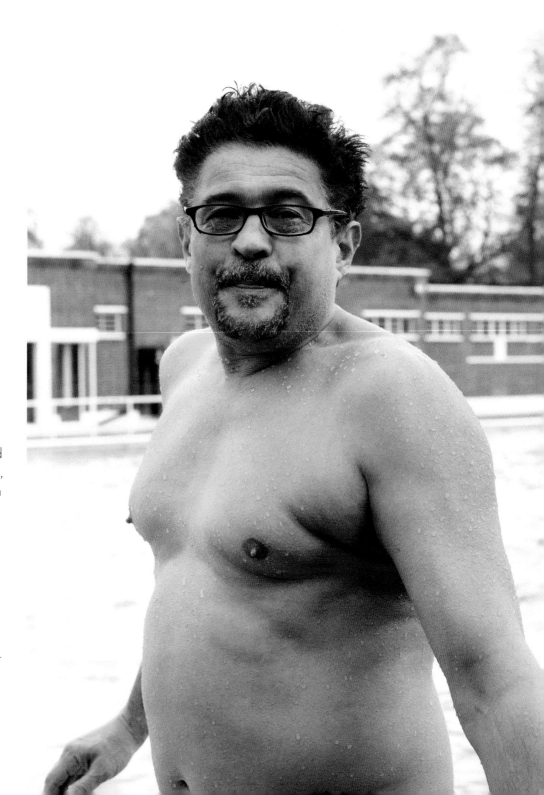

Chris Roberts
Not just the pool

Thing about cold water swimming at Brockwell Lido is that it's not just the pool.

For a start, there's the parks. Brockwell Park, London's most complete green space, is only the end of it. In the years I've been swimming at the lido, I've cycled either through or alongside other splendid examples of the Victorian Park, including Kennington, Myatt's Field and Ruskin, each, with their ever-changing treescapes, providing a teaser for the main event. Kennington once had its own lido, Myatt's Field has a fountain and stone cats that stare down sternly from Calais Road while Ruskin has,

alongside some of the best views over the city, a children's paddling pool and ponds that give rise to the Earl's Sluice, one of London's lost streams. Closer in to Brockwell is the better known River Effra that churns in front of the lido under Dulwich Road.

Many rivers to cross, one might say, with a nod back across Dulwich Road to the studio of Brixton's grandfather of dub poetry, Linton Kwesi Johnson, nestled, appropriately, near the cluster of streets known as poet's corner. Thing is though, it's not just the parks, or even the poetry from John Ruskin to Kwesi Johnson, there is also the sky. Viewed from the lido approach on winter mornings, the sun rising from behind Dulwich—or Tuscany, as one fanciful politician described the area—lends a suitably rural touch to south London. Once in the pool, it can be spied through the turnstile, or tipping over the wall, gradually claiming the pool side for light and burning off the damp settled chairs. On misty days, it's just a glimmer; on others, it shares the sky with the fleeing moon or makes shapes among the passing clouds.

On clear days, jetstreams cross the sky and invite thought of arrivals and departures. But for most people in the lido in winter, they are exactly where they want to be and exactly the moment they want to be there. However, it's really not about being in your favourite place, because we share it. Not just with other swimmers, but with the wildlife. Etta Duck and

Bob Maurice Mallard, whose arrival every spring marks that season, just as the geese flypasts and frantic squirrel activity mark the autumn. Smaller birds nest in the surrounding ivy and creeper, while wagtails dance the pool side and bubble gum-footed feral rock doves peck the surround for crumbs. Even these least-loved of London's birds appear majestic when soaring across the pool, so the blue of the water reflects nobly on their grubby undercarriages. Another unloved flying species which pass over head are the chattering Hendrix parakeets forever quarrelling their way across the park.

It would be unkind too to ignore the crows increasingly visible as the foliage drops in autumn. Leaves twitch their way into the pool after switching green to burn to crisp, to gone: each day, a slightly altered vista can be seen of the

pool surround from the calm waters. The leaves are the most visible sign of change in the landscape, as rain can come at any point and, if you are already in the pool, is as welcome and as right as, well, rain. The cold advances like a tide, though, in steps and stages. Temperatures, air and water drop at different rates, then steady before falling again. As single figures are reached, toes are nipped, hands gripped and people mutter about 'two hat' days.

Because it's not just about the pool, it's about the people. There is probably a ballet to be written, composed, choreographed, whatever it is one does with ballet, around how lido citizens prepare to enter the water. These dancers, boxers, divers and boppers, those plungers, dippers, waders and slippers, some of whom

shimmy, headstand, clap or flap like terrible plucked birds before entry. One day in mid-November, a figure in a white hat and large black goggles emerged steaming from the poolside caravan sauna like a 1950s Sci Fi monster, only to douse himself in the waters and become human again. Then there are the, largely silent, watchers in the yellow. The guards of life in their raised chairs who must find it funny and absurd, but they, like the rest of us, see great beauty in the natural world around the pool and the wealth of humanity in it.

Oh and yes the water is cold, it wakes you up and, like the Sci Fi monster, makes you human again to talk and sit and share breakfast. Every day before 8.30 in the morning when I get to work, I've had this world already.

Chapter 5

Helen Milstein 79
Life saver
Geraldine Martick 80
It makes you glad to be alive, swimming
Chris Bennett 82
A life in cold water (apologies to Tim Krabbe)
Julie Reynolds 84
A water-filled, painted blue hole in the ground
Valerie Lambert 90
Cold water conversations
Carolyn Weniz 92
A duck to water
Dave Woodhead 94
It's the wide-eyed wonder and drop-jawed
astonishment of my offspring

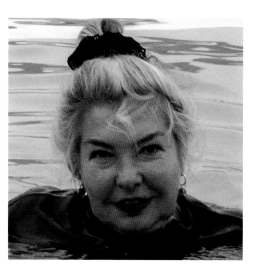

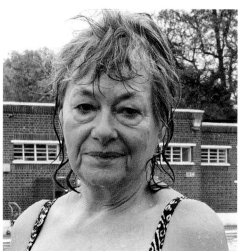

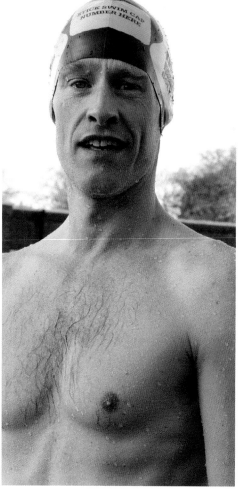

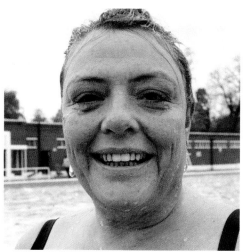

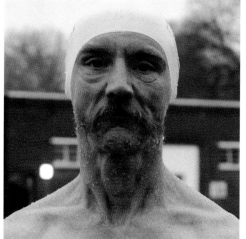

Lynda Laird

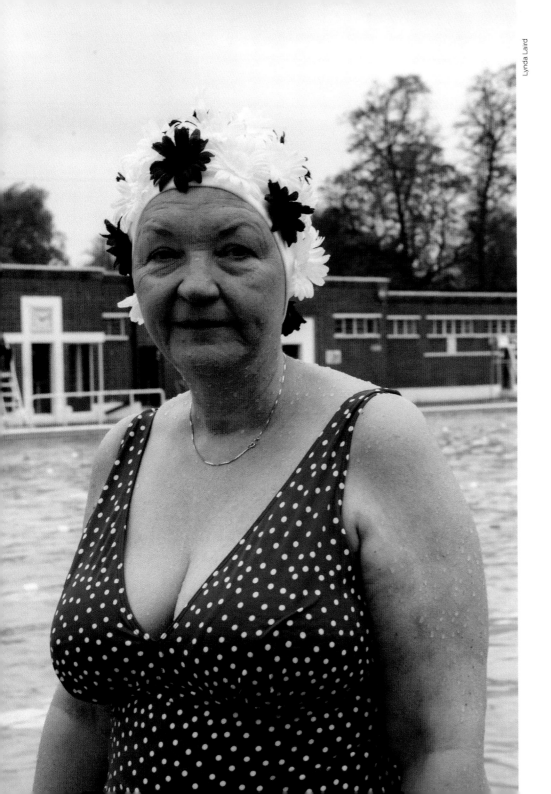

Lynda Laird

Helen Milstein
Life saver

Immersing yourself in the pool,
When the crowds have all gone away
And the skies are increasingly grey;
It's a perfect way to keep cool
Through the cares of the following day.

As the dark of the winter descends
And your mind feels invaded by night,
When just getting up is a fight,
It's a blessing to sit with your friends,
Sharing coffee and laughter and light.

If you feel that your life is a mess,
Don't sit in your house feeling gloomy,
The pool in the winter's quite roomy,
Your problems will bother you less
And the voice in your head is less boomy.

In short, it's a boon for your soul
And your body, you'll never turn back.
No more will your world seem so black,
When flooded with blue is your goal,
You'll be certain you're on the right track.

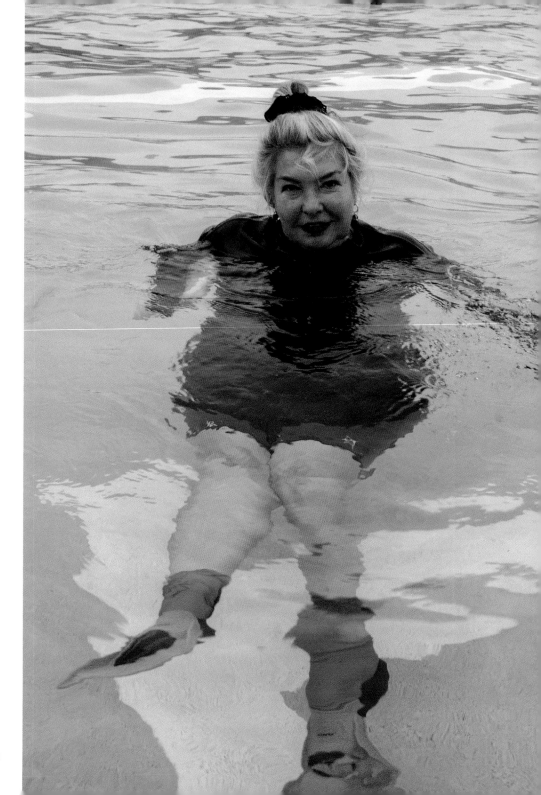

Geraldine Martick
It makes you glad to be alive, swimming

I learned to swim with my school in Dulwich baths. The clearest memory is struggling to learn breast stroke and despairing, thinking to myself that I would never get it, then one day suddenly I could do a length. Well, that was the start of it, a lifelong pursuit of immersion in municipal pools.

My first time in Brockwell Lido was at about 9 or 10 years old. Children were allowed to run free then and I don't remember any adults being with us kids. The sensation of the day was a woman wearing a leopard-print bikini. She sent an electrifying ripple through the crowded terraces and people craned their heads for a glimpse of her as she walked to the café. Since that first day, the Lido has always held a special place in my heart and it still always feels like a treat to be there. Having bought my first flat in Brixton many years later, I started swimming on my way to work. It was handy, being on my way to Herne Hill Station. I felt bereft when they closed it for a few years. Compelled to swim, I went further afield: Chelsea baths, Marshall Street baths, in Soho, the Oasis in Covent Garden. Even though the Oasis was open air, it didn't match up to the memory of the Lido with the trees around it and the birds swooping overhead.

The Lido was rescued from being turned into a carpark by the young lifeguards, Casey McGlue and Paddy Considine. They, with their friends Dog

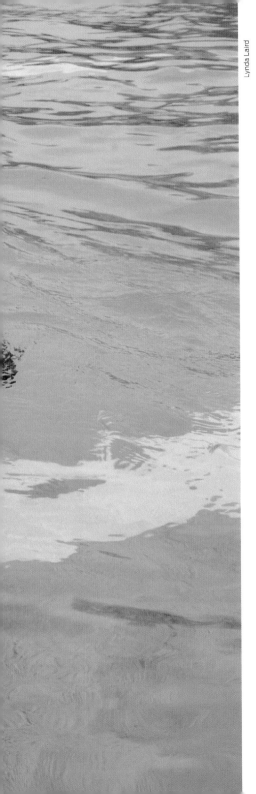

Lynda Laird

and Dangerous, turned it into a vibrant but laidback pool. 'Brixton Beach' they called it and they held extra enjoyments like Friday night barbeques and floodlit swimming. It was wonderful spending whole days lidoing at the weekends, instead of just swimming in the mornings. Dangerous used to make the announcements over the tannoy if there were problems in the car park. The whole place would erupt in laughter at his pronouncements in his broad Jamaican style.

I made most of my Brixton friends in those happy long summer days— including regular swimming companions. We would chat and swim our 10 lengths. Or swimming alone, watching

trees and the nesting birds in the dense ivy and wisteria on the walls. Looking at the clouds or up in the sky at the green parrots and the swifts.

Things change, of course, as things always do and the lease was awarded to Fusion. They built the gym and did it very well. I guess they had to make it financially viable and not so weather-dependent.

A few years ago, they started opening in the winter season. One enjoyed swimming until the end of October through the Indian summers in September. Then it was time to go indoors, Clapham Manor Street or Dulwich, my *alma mater.*

I had a sneaking envy of the

winter swimmers. Resolving to try and last a bit longer with a short wetsuit, in 2014, I made it to December 15 before being felled by flu.

My regular swimming didn't begin again until next April, as I lost my immunity to cold water. Autumn 2015, I had a flu jab, grimly determined to make it through the winter. The colder water slowly became more enjoyable. It was strange how elated I felt afterwards. A real natural high, 'endolphins', as Roger Deakin describes the feeling in his book, *Waterlog.* It really became even more addictive than regular swimming, no weather too foul to endure, who cares, if you are wet anyway? It is the magic of watching the seasons change as the

trees turn yellow and red then dropping their leaves and seeds in the water like an aquatic nature trail. The ducks when they join us in the water in early spring, sometimes with darling ducklings. The slow greening of the trees in March and then in April the blossom on the chestnuts.

Then, best of all, May, when the wisteria on the walls emits a cloud of sweet perfume over the terraces. It makes you glad to be alive, swimming.

Chris Bennett
A life in cold water (apologies to Tim Krabbe)

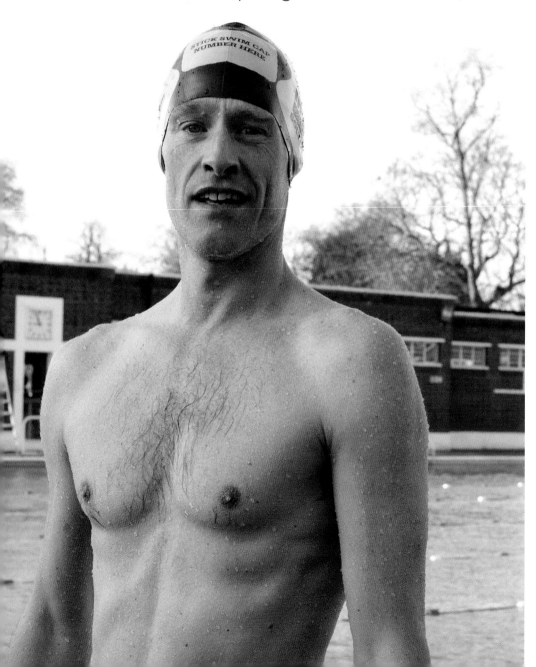

Lynda Laird

A boy leans back, spreads his arms along the warm stone weir edge, turns his face sunward and lets the cold water fall across his body.

The wrongness of being in the river pleases him as much as delicious relief from the searing 1976 heat: adults' orders to stay away overpowered by cool river water. Since he and his friends beat their way through cow parsley fields to duck beneath barbed wire and jump into the salmon ponds, the sun has sunk below green Devon hills. Close heat persists but light fades as mayfly gather above the surface of the water.

Young trout dart between his fingers, young friends dart from pond to pond in the salmon ladder's deep warm pools: six leaps warm the water before it rejoins the rest of the river, running in broad, rapid shallows nearby. The level is low, dried by summer drought and depleted by the factory leat, which draws water close by. Cold water cascades through salmon ponds, across the weir and on towards town. Children's cold water fear keeps them away from the leat and a deep elbow below the weir, but for a short few days the salmon ponds tame the cold water. As a young trout settles in his hand, the boy closes his fingers around its slippery body, holding it fast. He starts to call his friends to show off his catch but holds back. He feels the warm stone against his back, releases

the parr, lifting it to safety up and over into the next pond. Freedom.

An adolescent stands on the bridge drunk with excitement and cider. The dark cold water flows far below the bridge as two friends teeter on the handrail. He resists the calls to join them, embarrassed by his cowardice and conventionality. The water looks deep, but the fear of the drop and hidden depths hold him back. Brave fools are urged along to where the water is known by locals to be deep, a vortex? A dark, bottomless pit. Fear is written on young faces as the cold water vies with the desire to please the breathy, plump girls watching on. One jumps shrieking into the air, the adolescent feels the dread as he watches the body disappear below the water. It emerges laughing and whooping as a second, a third denim-clad figure falls through the air, their fear of the cold water suspended by alcohol and a desire to please. More climb to jump, but the adolescent's fear of the cold water's unknown is greater than his need to please. The cider's power insufficient, he cannot jump. Regret.

Two young men shiver as they tumble along the ice cold water on a makeshift raft towards the sea. Their fear of the cold water was suspended by ladders and inner tubes lashed together and testosterone-fuelled self-belief. Rawness of cold water has humbled them. They fight to keep their legs out of chill, swirling, splashing flow as they are dragged, helpless, ever-closer to trees hovering above powerful, swift, deep channels. A large immovable branch nears, they are thrown into the cold water and an unstoppable flow pins them to a bark wall. One young man holds his friend's head above the water for a few anxious moments as the cold water attempts to take his breath away. They panic as the wet icy wall holds them fast. Threat of drowning forces them to dive beneath the surface to be flushed downstream by the cold current. Their shivering numbness is suspended by the relief at being free. Fear.

A student watches his breath condense against a becalmed sailboard's boom as the reservoir shore drifts away. December days are short, light is fading. The confident sailor gave no heed to the cold water and tacked across the mirror towards a stone turret. Morning's gentle breeze, so easy to navigate, is now gone. He smiles with regret at overconfidence in his ability to stay aboard. As his hands slow with increasing cold he moves to de-mast and paddle back to the cold water's edge and a waiting, laughing crowd. He slips, falling theatrically into a brutally cold enclosure, the mirror breaks. The stinging cold of the lake tears his breath away and makes his body burn. He scrambles back aboard and paddles for shore,

his respect for the cold water renewed. Embarrassment.
Foam collects in cauliflower blooms in the rock pools that fringe a Newquay beach. An uncle and two young nephews wait by the cold water's edge to fulfil a dare laid down at Christmas celebrations some nights before. They are held back by the fear of the cold water; powerful surf pounds the sand. The dare's enormity is compounded by reality, crashing waves for the youngsters and crashing hangover for their older companion. As they move closer, mums shout warnings, building fear for the cold water, brothers goad a hungover show-off. Three figures walk to the cold water's edge as a family gathers behind, cameras in hand. They link hands and run, a screaming line engulfed by the waves.
As cameras flash, a moment of family history, to be recounted for years to come, is created. Achievement.

Two young boys spurred on by family stories gather on a New Year's Devon shore. Youngsters, eager to re-enact the cold water dare they have heard of so many times. They plead to a father. Feigning reluctance, he grudgingly agrees, relishing the water. Inside, his delight and pride swells. Harsh cold grips them all as they stand on the sand. The biting cold drives them on, they run into the sea and wrestle a few strokes of crawl. As the father swims to

warm himself he remembers the raw cold and respect for the water. He looks up fearful for his sons. Two boys dash back onto the sand. A grandmother's promise of a towel and hot chocolate, with all the trimmings, is too strong an excuse to stay in. Marshmallow heaven and a family tradition is born. Bonding.

A triathlete looks at his white, bloodless feet against the concrete reservoir slipway. His body is ready for the long swim to come, but the vast expanse of water and chill air renew his fear of the deep cold. A sea of wetsuited athletes stand in near silence, earlier banter stolen by the cold's reality. Pioneers enter the water. Their capped heads are lost from view below the white horses kicked up from the surface and they return to the safety of the slipway. Some emerge and walk away, not prepared to face the cold any longer. Huge marker buoys sway in the wind as the neoprene wave merges, gasping, with the water. A siren sounds, water bubbles, thousands of feet and hands spring into life. Wetsuits grapple in the crush. Strong arms thread into the distance in a long white line, the slow and timid hold back or move wide. Blue caps bobbing in clear water. As the metres build, the cold of the water eats away at their strength. Arms cramp, fingers become lost appendages, the water slipping through numb palms prolonging the agony. The relief of land finally comes, wetsuits

stagger and stumble on the painful concrete. Wetsuits fall, helpers sit some down and throw foil capes around their shoulder. Others look back with grim respect as they race on. Respect.

A man pushes through the lido turnstile to the edge of the tamed cold water. Its art deco containment misleadingly belies its biting cold. At first, his body arched to suck in air as he entered its crystal clear cold blueness. Its bite burning his skin, leaving his legs purple, his fingers a bloodless white, dizzy. But the tame water has befriended the man. Accustomed to the cold and seasons changing to warm, he visits the water often. A cold wet friend to commune with when he wishes. His worries and fears left with his crumpled clothing in the dry brick building. Those early frantic winter fights with the water are over. He is embraced by it, drawing himself through with long pulls as his friend supports his weight. As the seasons change, the water's mood will cool, its harshness returning, but the man returns to his friend still. Sometimes for distance, sometimes for speed, always for pleasure. When the weather is warm, he even stops and thinks, at the deep end, under the diving board. He leans back, spreads his arms along the warm stone pool edge, turns his face sunward and lets the cold water fall across his body.

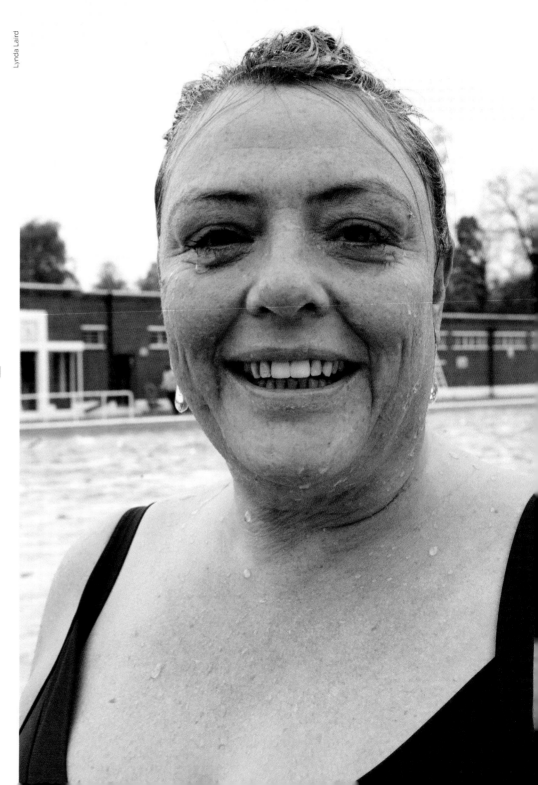

Lynda Laird

Julie Reynolds
A water-filled, painted blue hole in the ground

I first came to Brockwell Lido when I moved to London in 1994. Back then, it was wickedly uninhibited. Drinking and drugs were as much a part of the landscape as jiggling bare breasts and the snuggly fitting Lycra that encased the undulating bulges and mounds. Sunny days would result in feverish excitement at the prospect of a day with friends at 'Brockwell Beach', with a picnic, wine and papers. Getting there early to claim a good spot for the day, in the right part, was essential in showing who you identified with and how much you liked to party. Over the years, the Lido became a place that I visited not just to have fun but also to contemplate, to grieve and to heal.

Some 20 years after my first dip, I bought a season ticket and swam through the summer. I knew that I had to swim a lot to make it pay for itself and to feel like I was getting something for free. I also knew that I was in a place in my life where I would need to

find something therapeutic that went beyond talking once a week. When my world seemed to be collapsing, I swam through the black hole and found another universe. Here I found that I could leave my pool of despair and tap into my fountain of optimism. In this place, I can harness something that lets me be my most magnificent and powerful, or let go to be the tiniest, most insignificant wave in the biggest of oceans. The water has a magic. The colder it gets, the more powerful the magic gets, so I swam through the autumn and winter too.

April 20
Looks like a Lido morning. Sun out birds sing. 26 lengths felt like I was just getting going. So lovely. 3 kites dance like jelly fish in the sky above the park.

April 27
Lido and garden centre. Ground hog day.

May 15
Another lovely Lido swim. Pool shared with 3 ducks. Swifts swooping and spinning. Wagtails wagging, parakeets squawking, even the humble street pigeon's underbelly and wings are electric blue. A good way to wash the day away. Have to watch out for the wetsuits: I was like a seal being pursued by killer whales yesterday.

May 21 Too tired to swim today. Trying to build up from 3 times a week to 5. I find I like it when it's not so sunny; it's more peaceful with fewer people. I hope I can keep going through the winter. Could go on about snapped leg and the ducking stool, but thought I wouldn't.

June 20 In Lido Café with a crafty beer after a swim.

June 25 Lovely swim

August 19 London is chilly, swim this morning so stunning. Being eye-level in the water as the light dances on it is mesmerising. I can see everything and nothing. Mind clearing and filling at the same time. And I noticed the feel of the water as I move through it.

September 23
Grey London morning brightened by the oasis that is the Lido. In here, white clouds as curly as a lamb's wool float across the blue sky directly above. A scattering of wisteria still remains among the reddening leaves rippling in the breeze. The sun popped out for a while, but is mostly obscured, a light powdery yellow, looking more like the moon in the hue of the cloud. 20 lengths. A shower and out into a rainburst in the real world.

September 26
Even greyer London morning, no curly poodle-haired clouds or rising sun shining out. Just a blanket of grey. The heaviness of the sky was reflected in my slow 'moving through treacle' swim. It feels colder. I am aware of my skin tightening, goose bumps rising, hairs standing up and and an ever so slight tingling in my fingers and toes, but I

like that. A twist of the knee yesterday meant had to fashion a stroke that didn't use my right leg, leaving me with straight unmoving legs trailing behind me like enormous uncooked sausages. It is the first time I have doubted that I can keep going all winter. This could be grim on a winter's morning. Then five pigeons swooped over, underwings still reflecting the bright blue of the pool despite the grey day. A smile cracked through my grimace and 20 lengths are done. Someone in the shower asks me if I will swim through the winter. Indeed, I will, I find myself saying with certainty

September 29 My zen and usually serene smile was disrupted by two men, contorted faces panting and grunting up my rear, each trying to reach the end before the other—practically came up my back: no pun intended. All that grunting! Really? Took a while to recapture my former meditative state.

October 1 Heavy clouds loomed and the sky was again a dense grey, even

the noise of the airplanes took on a new muffled sound. Then the rain started. What joy! The impact of each rain drop caused a mass of rhythmic circular oscillations on the surface of the pool and I am part of a spectacular otherworldly yet natural psychedelic event. I did not want to get out. And all before work.

October 3 The sky was blushed pink with billowing clouds radiating a weird nicotine yellow. As the sun began to rise, the dancing tree tops were illuminated gold. The pool rippled with yellows and pinks. The quiet only broken by the lapping of the water and the rumble of the occasional plane. As I swam towards the sun, it was momentarily captured in the centre of the turnstile, glowing and framed. If I had not been in that exact part of the pool at that exact time of day and year, or had a cloud passed by, or my eyes been closed I would not have witnessed the time that the golden sun was caged, nor its gentle escape.

October 4 Sleep more, or

swim. Sleep-swimming: maybe I can do both. Ask the dog who ate them. Dogs are rubbish at telling lies. Cats on the other hand.

October 7 Pool temperature has dropped by 3 degrees since Sunday. 15.3 now, can see my breath with every exhale.

October 8 Getting ready for Lido in the dark is weird. Yesterday was amazing. Another noticeable drop in temperature and the sky as dark as raven wings. Pounding rain on water gave another spectacular display, the rain hitting so hard it sends millions of diamond topped droplets springing up. Can't believe how lucky I am.

October 9 First in the pool this morning. A huge moon remains in the sky, to be joined shortly after by a beautiful sun throwing golden light shimmering across the water. What I initially thought was a lonesome star's fading light was in fact the underbelly of a distant plane catching the early sun. Glorious.

October 10 Wow, this morning was so beautiful. I am the first swimmer again. Cold and crisp with a steely blue sky, chilly, calm still water. I swim

towards the moon at one end and the sun coming up at the other. Just breath-taking. I cannot think of a better way to start the day.

October 13 A dirty wet morning. Heavy greyness oppressing down. No hint of sunshine. No birds swooping across the pool. Only a neck-less crow, looking like an undertaker, his head sunk down into his wings like the collar of an overcoat, watched miserably from the roof of the pump room.

I finally got through to one of my fellow swimmers that my name is not Jenny. He had been greeting me with a 'Morning, Jenny' for almost 3 weeks before I even realised he was talking to me. When I did realise, I kept telling him that I am not Jenny, but he did not seem to hear.

Although slightly embarrassed, he says that he is glad that I told him, as someone has been calling him Gerald for the past 5 years; the person has called him that for so long he hasn't got the heart to say that that's not his name. He told me what his name is, but I have forgotten. Maybe I should call him Gerald.

October 16 Beautiful morning. Clear blue sky with a whisper of cloud. Low damp patches of steamy mist hover

above the grass in the park in a mini beast fog.

A small half-moon the colour of a mouldy segment of lemon eerily seems to follow me up and down the pool, as the sun glitters through the trees. Birds sing, crows caw and bright green parakeets swoop and squawk. Airplanes glide through the sky with underbellies looking like ancient masks.

October 27 Early this week, had cloud-bruised sky and wind that whipped trees, sending leaves swirling into the choppy-watered pool. The fading crescent moon like a lash-less eye blinked out of the bright blue cloudless morning sky yesterday. A wagtail landed at the side inches away from my face eyeing me with a tilted head and bobbing his tail.

October 29 Yesterday's spectacularly bright retina-burning morning was replaced and heavy grey cloud now fills the atmosphere. No blue to be seen. The pool is warmer at 14.6 and I had it to myself for a while. I like to calmly glide through the water enjoying the quiet stillness feeling the cold of the water and the vaguest rumble of the unseen airplanes. Calmness halted by 3 men. One making a fuss about the cold, another thrashing about

like he was drowning and another in tiny speedos, a swimming cap and enormous rubber gloves. Looked like a naked mole rat. 22 lengths. Got out because my top lip was numb.

November 4 Pool temperature dropped from 14.6 to 13.2. Beautiful crisp sunny morning. Some trees are now naked, others seem to have lost very few leaves and others are left with just a few swaying on their branches like a last fan dance.

Sun came up, forming golden ripples across the pool; for a moment, it was reflected off the pump room window, casting a vanilla slice yellow strip down the other end of the pool. Bloody glorious. 24 lengths. 40 minutes. Corned beef legs for a while after. I am told at 12 degrees hands and feet hurt. Thinking about putting my swimming cap on and maybe invest in some gloves to give me otter hands.

November 5 Another wonderful morning sunny and cold. A world of aqua blue and gold.

November 6 Frosty morning. Filled with excitement and trepidation as I cycled past frost-covered cars on the way to Lido. Spectacular sunrise over park as I arrived. Mist like dry ice floating above the pool. Air temperature 4, pool 11.6. First couple of lengths felt cold, patches of skin felt like salted grazes, head freeze like gulping an icy cocktail. For a moment it felt like my skin was being separated from my forehead and peeled back. Then it settled down. Amazing swim through fog. Swam into a rocket from last night's display, picked it up and gave it to the lifeguard, who asked, 'Did you find it in the pool?' No, I said, I brought it with me. 3 lengths alone. I bloody love it. I am so privileged to have found this amazing watery world.

November 10 Glad to be back in the water! Another lovely morning moon-and-sun combination. Crows dance on tall buildings, magpies jumping on rooftops and a small murmuration of starlings doing acrobatics. Pool 11.2. I think I am made for coldwater swimming—some distant evolutionary code still present in my genetics. Someone asks, 'Why do you smile so much? Are you mad?'

November 15 This week's swimming has seen more spectacular mornings. Yesterday was so dark with moody fierce clouds. Then the rain came lashing down onto the pool it was like swimming through watery stalagmites. It is impossible not to be in the moment,

the experience and to feel invigorated and ready to take on the world. A good job, what with the new crack den in the upstairs flat and all the chaos that is emerging from it. I woke on Thursday morning and peeked out of the window into the morning darkness and saw what I thought was snow on the steps. My excitement was replaced by fury to find the contents of a foam-filled mattress making a junkie Hansel and Gretel trail to said den. Front door onto street propped firmly open for easy access. Only thing it lacked was a blood spurt sign saying 'drug den this way'. Most surprised not to have found a herd of Camberwell's finest waxy-faced, blank-eyed, buffalo-breathed addicts corralling through the door as I left for the Lido.

November 17 Clouds turn from dark grey to the colour of a wood pigeon.

November 18 Poor new boy puts his toes in, then promptly walks away before coming back for another try. Looked like he was going in from a high board, such was the fear. I tell him it's lovely once you get in. Of course, this is just an opinion and one he did not share, judging by his reaction on getting in and his quick exit.

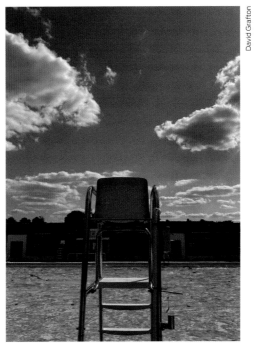

David Grafton

November 21 Pool rapidly heading for single figures, temperature dead on 10. 18 lengths; each felt like my skin was shrinking like wool jumper in the tumble dryer. Weirdly enjoyable.

November 28 There must have been some weird thermals over south London this morning. Shakespeare Road was a blizzard of golden spiralling leaves like all the ones remaining on the trees had waited for the same moment to let go of the trees. A woman walked towards me arms outstretched, both of us laughing in amazement that we had witnessed this. From the pool, I could see about 50 gulls gliding, soaring and

swooping over the park, later to be joined by crows for a while. Then the murmuration of starlings joined in for a while before landing in a skeletal tree. The wagtails jumped and bobbed at the side of the pool chirping happily, even a flock of ducks did a fly by. On one of my turns at the pool side, I was greeted by an almost cylindrical flurry of leaves and sycamore spinners spiralling down into the water. Beautiful and breathtaking.

December 3 Yesterday morning was damp, just dank, not really even like rain, more like cold perspiration under a dark grey blanket.

Today though was one of those cold, clear mornings where the wind cuts through you a bit. Beautiful clouds like ripened peaches and pigeon plumage floating across crisp blue sky, keep me watching and smiling in the moment. Pool 8.9 When I first got in, I had weird stigmata-ish pains in my hands and feet like they were being pierced with a very sharp object. Very odd. Went away after about 6 lengths—Satan must have caught me.

Bitter wind swept across the pool from the café side, making the water choppier than usual and blowing spray in my ear. 18 lengths and corned beef feet and bosoms, but still loving it.

December 6 Frosty morning. By far the coldest yet. Clear Blue sky, huge golden sun. Frost around the pool, water temperature 7.5, gloriously cold on the hands and feet. It's like it's meant to be when I am in here. A heightened sense of being.

I stay for 25 minutes, but the swimming is slow, only 12 lengths. I worry why I do not feel cold, but at the end I dive under the water a couple of times, skimming my belly along the bottom of the pool. The head freeze is like a mouth full of popping candy. As soon as I get to the changing rooms, I want to go back in. I resist, in case I am delirious. No corned beef skin, no ill affects. Just left wanting more.

December 9 A stunningly beautiful morning. Amazing light. Both moon and sun visible. But you know it's going to be cold when they have gritted and salted around the pool.
6.3. Toes and fingers hurting and feeling like concrete. Face feeling like it's having a million paper cuts. A painful strange delight. 10 lengths in 20 minutes. Brrrrr

December 10 Splendid morning. Bright. Last night's winds evident in Myatt's Field Park, dead wood, twigs and branches scattered about. Moon looking glorious in crisp blue sky with burnt orange sunrise. Air temperature not as cold as yesterday, it didn't feel as biting in the pool, even though it is still 6.3. Body more adjusted, 12 lengths in 20 mins.

December 16 Arriving at Lido this morning. A chilly 6.3. Body felt like it was being stabbed with a million needles for first 2 lengths, but the amber glow of the sunrise soon distracted me. A seagull soared over the pool; the sun caught its underwing, making it golden. 10 lengths in 20 mins. Happy.

December 22 A bit of a grey morning with dark clouds racing across the grizzly sky. I greeted the man who feeds the pigeons in Myatt's Field Park. I always try to cycle slowly past so as not to cause the birds to get the fear and start frantically fluttering about my head … It never works. The man wishes me a merry Christmas and his friend waves his crutch.
The pool is busy and choppy, lots of waves, spray and wind in my face and hair, lovely.

No evidence of the creatures that left the enormousness shits on the poolside at the deep end last week. Possibly geese, but do they just stand shitting, making a pile as big as a large dog? I don't know. Anyway, last week we were down to 6.3 in the water, but the warmer air temperature has put some heat into the pool and it is now a sizzling 8 degrees. 14 lengths, could have stayed in for much longer … Except I had to go to work.

Roll on Christmas Eve, when I can have a more leisurely swim before the frantic Xmas shopping/cooking …

December 27 Pool back down to 6.2 after Christmas day's 8.1. It is such a joy. 20 lengths on Christmas Day with a bit of diving and enjoying the winter sun, in for 35 minutes, no ill effects. Today just 12, finishing off with a couple of dives to the bottom of the pool for a head freeze. Warmed up in sauna afterwards, all followed by half-price coffee in Lido Café and home-made cake and biscuits brought by other swimmers. What better start to the day could there be?

December 28 Cold clear crisp morning sparkling with frost, perfect for … a swim

December 29 Cold, crisp icy weather: looks like a good day for … cycling out to see a deer's breath in Richmond Park … and a tasty lunch by a fire at a pub on the river … after my swim.

December 31 Another year gone – time, it's all relative.

There once was a collision
of dimensions,
that created cosmological extensions,
a universe began
with a very big bang
expanding complex theories
and tensions

Photo last sunrise and swim of the year

January 6 Bit of a grey morning. Felt colder than the 6.2 that was on the board, but it could just have been the choppiness.

January 9 Wake up considering the events going on in the world both close to home and across the sea with sadness and a heavy heart. Spectacular morning sky. Pool lovely 6.7 degrees. Only 10 lengths. Lovely little wagtail beady-eyed and pale yellow face fluffed up by the side of the pool waiting for some spray.

January 12 Insomnia and indigestion the frosted icing on a day that started with me dragging myself up and down the pool in a joyless manner, hoping my lack of enthusiasm is just a temporary New Year lull, followed by having a meeting about funding cuts, then having to push the bike home in the dark, pouring rain because I had a puncture.

January 14 Maintaining joy for swimming has been difficult this year. I spend much of my time anxious about the world and my place in it. Feeling bad about both what I have done and also what I haven't. My internal world becoming as complicated and tangled as the external one. I cannot find a place of inner calm or a way to soothe myself.

January 15 It falls back into place again, I am able to leave horrors, pain and anxiety of life and the world we live in somewhere—the cold changing rooms, perhaps—and the tightening, coiled-up spring of my mind and body starts to loosen. I can see beauty, even if it is just a fleeting moment.
It is perhaps that I see beauty more profoundly when I am cold and almost naked in a water-filled, painted blue hole in the ground. Perhaps my senses are heightened or numbed, but from here it seems uncomplicated to feel only what is here and now. The sky the water the light how they interact and how I am submerged in them I am reassured by their ever-changing familiarity. Contentment settles in.

January 22 Yesterday, back in the pool after missing almost a week. The infection in my back is finally shrinking

more like a white chocolate button than its previous lemon fondant fancy. Pool temp 4.6. First 2 lengths felt like my fingernails were being pulled out, before hands been jumped on. By 6 lengths it has settled down and my body adjusts. I find the cold reassuring.

January 23 Pool a chilly 3.7. Nearly skidded on icy footprints on the way in. A sensible 6 lengths with no ill effects

February 4 Water a toe-curling 3.5. Sun popped out for a short while to give glittery ripples, but otherwise grey.

February 7 Coughing up blood balls, hope I don't have consumption. Perhaps the holly waters will cure.

February 16 Yay, pool now open at 7.10. Pool a sizzling 5.1. There was a snake of wires twisting through the door, about 10 people around the pool with lights and cameras. A man pumps smoke across the pool to photograph a renowned woman swimmer. Yes, they do that at 7.35 in the morning.

February 17 Beautiful morning. I can almost feel the still sleepy breath of spring in the air. Sun rising throwing a liquid gold ripple along the lengths of the pool. Turning at the deep end, I swim into it cold and numbed by the

water but warmed and energised by the sun.
Like yesterday, I am the only person in the pool. Today is serene quiet and peaceful. I swim up and down, happily gathering good thoughts like a catfish on the seabed.

March 1 Always makes me happy to see that the ducks are back and visiting regularly.

March 7 Pool warming up now, it's a lovely 7 degrees. Been beautiful all week, every morning the sun has been sparkling on the water and I have had it mostly to myself. This won't last long. Soon the wetsuits will arrive.

March 8 Warm sunshine, cool water; feeling like a happy otter.

March 9 So bloody lovely to catch the morning sun before the clouds bring greyness.

March 10 The season has started. Changing rooms, a fetish club of rubber and wetness. People wriggling in and out of gear leaving it dripping on every available hook. Although I do like the rubber balaclavas. If this is allowed, there should be a nude day. Far less offensive and much less smelly.

March 12 Glorious morning. Makes

me so happy. Pool temp 9.1 warm sunshine and clear blue sky. I swim with only 2 others. Birds sing. A wobble (I know not the right terminology) of blue tits flutters from tree to tree chirping loudly. A crow fixes an existing nest in a still naked tree, but there is a hint of purple buds.

Valerie Lambert
Cold water conversations

Cold water conversations 1
3 May 2016
Varinka (musing sadly on Prince while breaststroking along): Are you a Prince fan?

Therese (swimming past): No, darling, I'm not interested in any music after the 1960s.

Next day, in the showers

Varinka: I think you'd like my partner, Freddie, he's got an encyclopaedic mind for all musical genres, and he loves music from the 60s *(mentally pictures him in Liverpool, where he went to uni)*.

Therese: Oh lovely! How nice to have a partner. I haven't had a boyfriend for ages. I'd love a nice partner to share things with. Has he got any single friends?
Varinka (conjuring to mind Freddie's only single friend): Er yes, he does ... but I don't think you'd like him. He has a lot of girlfriends, one after the other. He has a nice girlfriend at the moment, but it won't last. We saw him last week without his girlfriend and he bagged off early with a woman he'd only just met.

Therese: Maybe he hasn't met the right one yet.

Varinka: Mmm, it's a bit more complex. I've known him for years. I know the way he operates. Twenty years ago it was 'unattractive postgraduates': his words, not mine. Now it is mid-life, slightly worried academics mainly. You see he likes ... er, how do I put it? ... to feel a sense of his own prowess. He likes GRATEFUL SEX.

Therese: (disgusted) Uuuuuugh! Eeeeeew! Oh, ugh, how horrible!
Varinka: I know. I'm sorry; it is an insurmountable barrier.

Veronique (having just come in from car park): What?

Therese: Varinka's just told me that her friend likes GRATEFUL SEX. Eeeeeeeeew!

Varinka: Technically, he's Freddie's friend.

Hedda (removing swim cap): Isn't it a bit early in the morning for this subject?

Varinka (feeling a bit sorry and strangely disloyal): Well, he does have

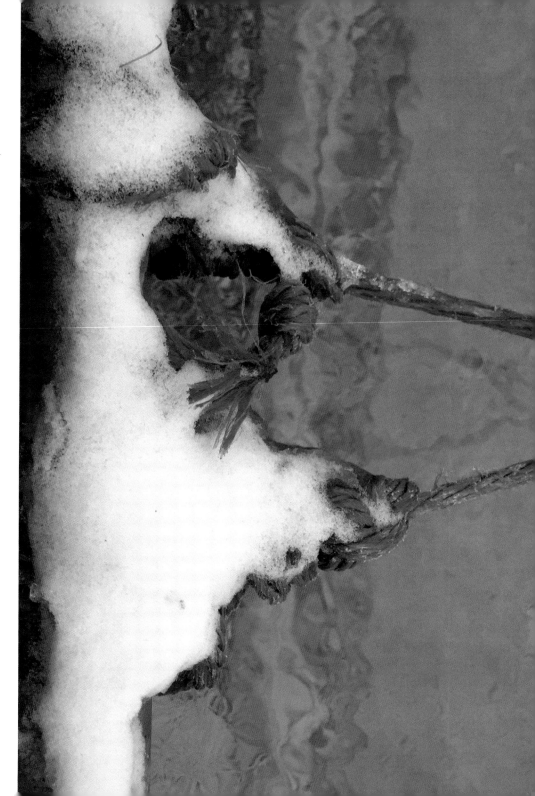

some pluses ... he is a good dancer and he has a good job, with a nice 1960s flat ...

Therese: The flat's the best thing so far.

Varinka: ... with excellent views over London ...

All: laughter and giggling.

Varinka (stifling laugh): ... and he's a town planner who genuinely cares about creating affordable homes.
Therese (laughing): We all do, darling! Do you think he'd like me in this? *(poses provocatively in tight, neoprene suit)*
Varinka: Yes! *(mimes taking a photo)*
Therese: Ha ha ... he'll do, then! *(disappears round corner towards pool)*

Cold Water Conversations 2

16 February 2016
In the changing room
Varinka (coming in from the pool): Brrr, Ellie, you're an experienced outdoors swimmer. What do you do when the temperature is lower than this?

Ellie: You'll get used to it. How long have you been swimming outdoors?

Varinka: Only since September: not counting childhood sea swimming ...

Ellie: Do you go back home much?

Varinka: Yes, I have to really ... but I like it. Sometimes I take a dip in the sea.

Ellie: Are your parents there?

Varinka: Yes ... *(thoughtfully)* they had a sort of crisis about two years ago and social services were called in, so I have to keep in touch with what is going on.

Ellie: Oh dear, did they have an accident?

Varinka: No, no ... it's quite difficult to explain, but they were leading life in a way that was unsustainable ... a kind of rock'n'roll lifestyle ... in their late seventies. I tried to talk to them for several years, but they ignored me ... then I didn't have to try any more because after several incidents, social services were alerted, and now women come in every day.

Ellie: And you visit regularly too.

Varinka: I notice things that the women don't.

Hedda (interested): What sort of things?

Varinka: Well, for example, I noticed when Dad began to cook for Mum, she wasn't eating what he made, and for a while she was wasting away. She just said a very definite 'No, thanks!' when

he took her tray in, and he accepted that ... because she had always been the boss in the domestic arena.
Hedda: Oh dear Lord, she could have starved while being served three meals a day!
Varinka: Yes, after 55 years of marriage, Dad didn't have a clue about what Mum liked to eat.

Ellie (who is a longtime friend of Hedda): That'll be you, Hedda.

Hedda (smiling acknowledgement): Yes ... true ... should I become *non compos mentis*, James might accidentally allow me to perish in a similar way.

Ellie (to Varinka): But they're OK now, your parents?

Varinka (smiling): Yes, they're OK ... they're muddling through. The young guns have become old guns, but they're fine, they're doing ... pretty well, for now!

Cold Water Conversations 3

16 June 2016
In the showers

Jaswinder (musing idly on feminine grooming): Var, do you remember when we found out about vajazzles?

Varinka: Yep, it was when *The Only*

Way Is Essex (TOWIE) was on TV; one of the girls was a beautician and she did them. She shaped, waxed and trimmed everything, then applied a little decoration just to the side.

Jaswinder: In tiny diamonds. It was such a shock to discover that those young women paid such detailed attention to that area.

Varinka: Difference between them and us, Jas. They're liberated ... different generation ... and seem to have visitors there, so it was worth it ... like a little WELCOME mat.

Louisa: Well I used to think it was polite just to pretend you hadn't noticed what was there. If *you* had a vajazzle, would it say 'WELCOME' in tiny rhinestones?

Varinka: I think I see myself as a little more mature and flirtatious ... perhaps 'KNOCK BEFORE ENTERING', ha ha, hahaha.
Jaswinder: Mine would say 'STAND CLEAR OF THE DOORS, PLEASE!'
All: laughing.
Varinka: What about you, Lou?
Louisa (with a disapproving look): 'CLOSED FOR REFURBISHMENT!'

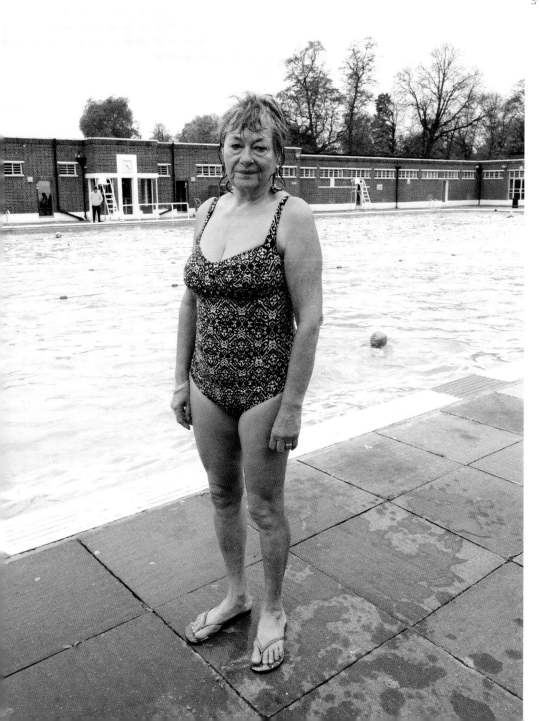

Lynda Laird

Carolyn Weniz
A duck to water

I so enjoyed swimming in the Lido in the summer, especially when it started staying open until the end of October, as the temperature invariably dropped and the lack of light curtailed evening swimming, but as the number of swimmers dwindled, so the camaraderie increased. The first opportunity for winter swimming in the Lido coincided with my retirement four years ago, so I knew there was a good chance of being able to stay the course through to April. I did, despite the weather in January, February and March being very cold and miserable throughout, with frequent snow showers into the second week of April.

The few who continued became true 'icicles', as a couple of times there was ice in the water.

I had never really thought about why I took to cold water swimming like 'a duck to water'. But, through discussing it with the other regular winter swimmers there that season, I realised that I had been initiated into it when I was at junior school. That was as a result of cold water swimming lessons at the local outdoor pool in Wiltshire, starting straight after Easter. Included were cold showers and a half mile or so shivering crocodile trek back. Some would regard it now as child cruelty! But it was not enough to put me off—I hated going in the heavily chlorinated, sweaty indoor pool for swimming lessons when I went to grammar school in a nearby town, in Somerset. Fortunately, as a special treat, for a few weeks each summer, we were able to go in the school's outdoor pool, which was no more than a glorified paddling pool. Long before going to secondary school, though, I would go to swim in a sizeable artificial lake on Longleat Estate with my family, every Sunday, and on hot days in the holidays and evenings in the summer. When Dad and Mum did not have to do their school cleaning jobs, we would have a hurriedly put together picnic—sandwiches, tea, biscuits and often stale homemade cake. If it was not long after the Corona man's delivery, a bottle of 'pop' and crisps might be included. The calm, deep, midge-infested water was a good way for me to escape from my squabbling younger brother and sister. In the height of summer, all I had to think about was avoiding the creepy, daily spreading mass of water lilies. The enormous depth never crossed my mind until a fellow school pupil was drowned when I was 15. Not long after, swimming in the lake was banned, but my parents thought the drowning was just the excuse the yacht club wanted so it could now race as much as it wanted all over the lake, without having to stay away from the swimmers.

During my subsequent 'hippy years', cold water swimming did not appeal, as it was not as cool as rock music, sex, drugs and politics. But, when I finished university and followed the hippy trail to California, cold swimming, which involved wilderness trips into the hills to search out cold water springs for respite from the heat of LA, regained its attraction. Of course, the trips were invariably accompanied by my hippy pursuits, minus the political activism, along with substantial supplies to fight off 'the munchies'.

Four years later and then extensive travelling in Greece, Turkey, followed by living in Iran offered few opportunities for cold water swimming. I remember standing by the Caspian in the spring, after the Revolution, longing to get in, but not willing to with all my clothes on, as etiquette now required.

Returning to the UK and living in Brighton, cold water swimming was now a part of my life, but despite Punk being on the wane, 'sex, drugs and rock and roll' and politics once again dominated my life and so limited my opportunities for getting in the sea.

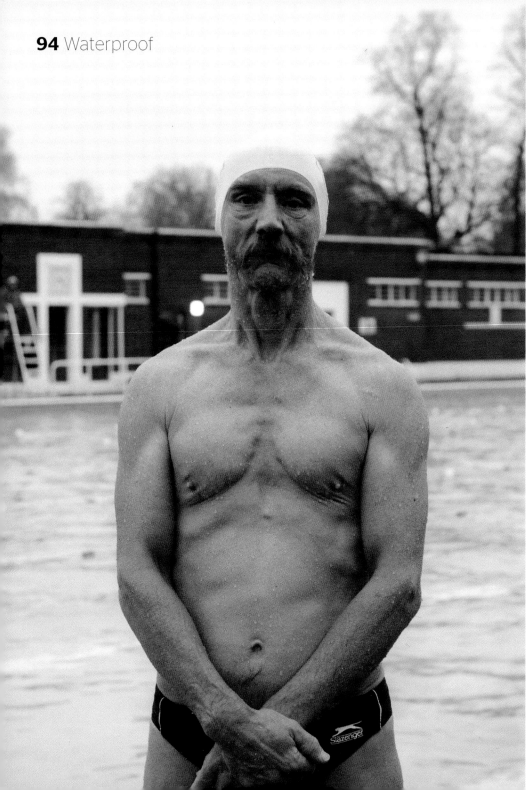

Lynda Laird

Dave Woodhead
It's the wide-eyed wonder and drop-jawed astonishment of my offspring

It's not the thrill of the first length, the temperature having dropped into single figures for the first time that season. It's certainly not the thrill of the sixteenth.

It's not the consequent release into the blood stream of such industrial quantities of exhilarating chemicals that a competitive cyclist could only marvel in awe and respect.

It's not the warmth of the shower or the changing room camaraderie.

It's not the scintillating discussion of minute fluctuations in the thermometer readings over the previous twenty-four hours.

It's not the cycling off into the outside world like a teeth-chattering, gibbering junkie leisurely appreciating the courtesy and considerate reticence of the south London rush hour car and van drivers as I head home.

Though any one of these would be reason enough to bring me to the health-giving spa waters of the Lido each morning, it is something else, more important still.

It's the getting home to the bosom of my family, to be surrounded by the admiration and respect of my offspring. It's the wide-eyed wonder and drop-jawed astonishment as I regale them with pithy anecdotes plucked from that morning's poolside chat.

'Daddy, daddy, do tell us this morning's water temperature,' they chorus.

It's then I come into my own, reeling off all the exciting detail of that morning's trip, my children barely able to contain their enthusiasm for the subject.

As my spouse places another hot coffee on the table before me, congratulating me on that morning's remarkable feat, I bask in the warmth of the scene (a sensation only equalled when pedalling south of Waterloo Bridge with a bellyful of the India Club's chilli bhajis).

It's then I reflect that, although pride comes before the fall, smugness will get you easily through to mid-March.

Chapter 6

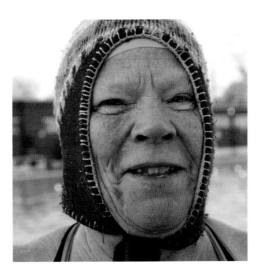
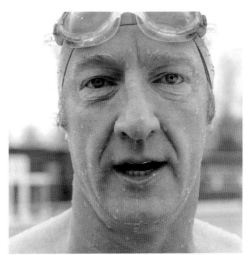
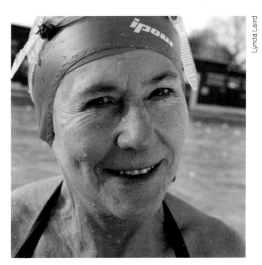
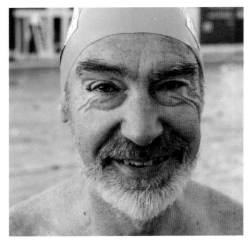
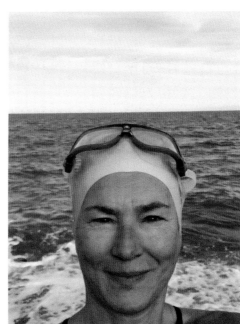
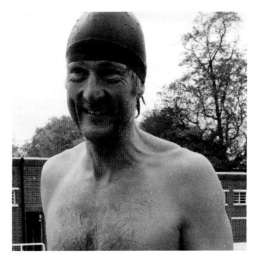

Lynda Laird

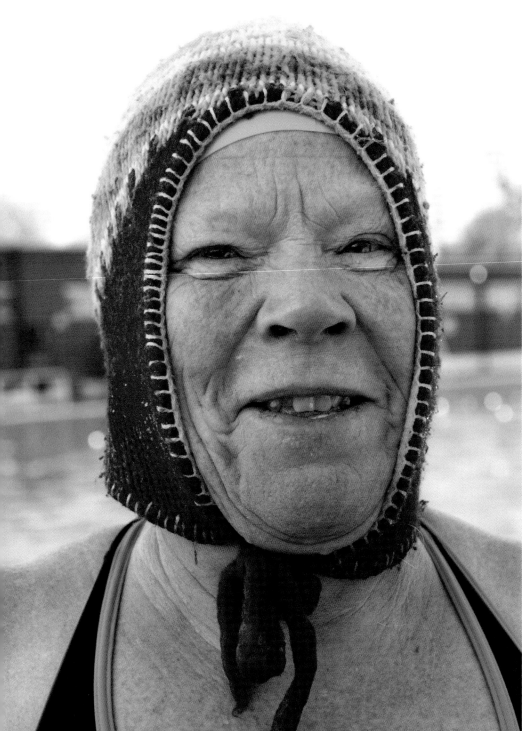

Lynda Laird

Marianne Atherton
A November swim

Apprehension as I cycle across the park—
How cold will it be?
Best not to look till after my swim ...
Outdoor change and a quick chat before heading down
the steps and into the water—
A familiar coldness and calmness takes over my body
and mind—
For a few minutes at least—all is well with the world.

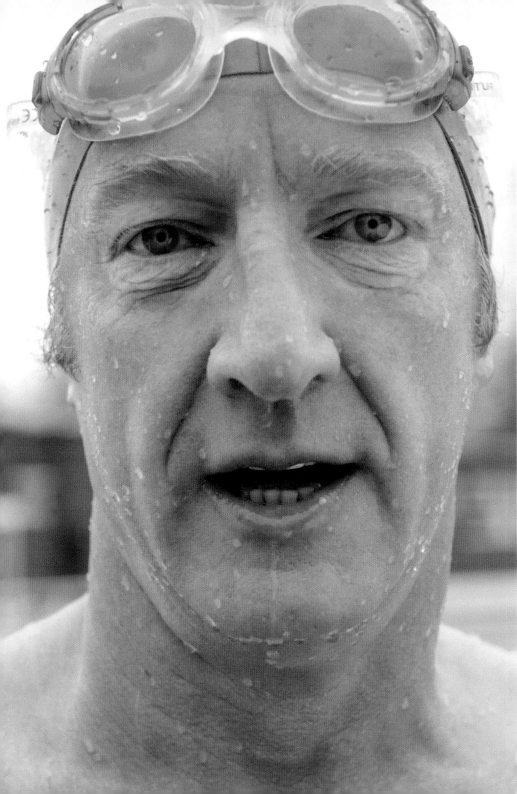
Lynda Laird

Steffan Rhodri
The colder the pool was, the more I was enjoying it

'Oh yes! I know you!', I shouted, pointing like a madman. I'd just returned to the Lido changing rooms after a shocking swim and my audible shuddering had amused an ex-colleague contentedly dressing there. It was late May 2015. I barely recognised or remembered him through the disorientated icy haze. The following May, the 16 or 17°C of the pool that day would seem balmy and I had become a card-carrying aficionado of Brockwell Lido; not only sporting my own defining cap of the self-styled and mercifully unorganised Brockwell Icicles, but having tasted my first synchronised swimming session to boot. The Lido had become an unexpected and magnetic haven for me.

As an actor, I've spent more than 15 years coming back and forth to London to work from my home in Wales. It's often been a lonely place, and at times my life here has been confined to work and spending time with the people I meet at it. I've stayed several times in digs close enough to

have visited the Lido: West Norwood, Tulse Hill, Nunhead ... But the two or three occasions I'd ventured had been, as for many visitors, limited to hot summer days in school term time when a refreshing dip in relative peace was guaranteed. But that May of 2015 brought me to new digs at the Somervilles on Croxted Road, Herne Hill, and my life was about to take a turn.

After that initial shocking day, I bought a swimming cap and already sensed the beginnings of an obsession. My addictive personality makes these obsessions very familiar: get all the gear, make big promises, go hell for leather for a couple of weeks, then pack it all in just as quickly. Except I haven't packed this in.

The South Wales valleys of my childhood were dotted liberally with outdoor pools, as much a part of many villages or towns as the Welfare Hall and library, and often paid for in the same way, through funds donated by workers:

coal miners, steelworkers or (as in the history of my lower Swansea valley home) tin and copper workers. I see now with nostalgic hindsight how we took them for granted: Morriston, my own home town; Clydach, a few miles north, where my gran and aunties lived; Ystalyfera, deeper into the coal field and a mining area until the 1980s, where I went to my Welsh language secondary school. Each of these had a run-down, faded, but beautifully austere outdoor pool. We never referred to these as a 'lido', which we always pronounced in the Italian way 'lee-do' (I still find it hard to adjust to the London version of 'lie-do'): 'Lido' was reserved for the grander and more deserving Afan Lido leisure complex near the beach beyond Port Talbot steelworks, a mammoth of post-war optimism for the beleaguered workers of that town. By the 1970s and 1980s of my childhood, it's remarkable that these outdoor pools survived at all: only opened on the warmest days of the summer months, sporadically understaffed by bored teenage lifeguards, presumably seconded from

the more comfortable indoor facilities nearby. They accurately represent the nationwide speedy decline and disappearance of these wonderful resources, and we all partook in their demise through ignorant neglect. I was late to learn to swim and so my own attendance at these outdoor pools was limited, like most of my peers, to splashing around and in breaking most of the famous retro wall signs' prohibitions: I don't remember smoking at poolside till a bit older and 'heavy petting' was a much-imagined future fantasy, but 'ducking' and 'bombing' were certainly on the cards, as well as the more benign 'diving' and 'shouting'. I was probably 10 by the time a crash course at the Swansea indoor baths rid me of the dreaded float and this late start has always affected my confidence in the water. But as age has caught up, knee injuries which ended my running and thorough ennui which restrict my gym attendance have left swimming as my main form of exercise.

The 50 yards of Brockwell intimidated

at first. But I'd tried Tooting once or twice as well and the 100 yards there positively terrified. So I persevered. I may well have continued to come every morning just for the swimming. But if the pool had been empty or if everyone hurried off after showering, the experiment might have been another on the list of middle-aged obsessions dropped by the wayside, along with the violin, motorbike, horse riding and accordion (I kid you not). But it wasn't, and they didn't.

Bringing breakfast was probably the key. A large tub of muesli set on the bench outside the Café became the entry fee to a wonderful circle of eccentric, intelligent, brave, intriguing comrades. First, David and Sara and their bizarre pre-swim rituals and synchronised dive, then Guy, followed by Peter S, Katie, Peter B, Maureen and soon a whole host of beautiful souls. I think it was Peter S who broke my anonymity by recognising me from a TV show I'd done. This gave me some instant notoriety and further reason to converse, as well as my shared Welsh

roots and the Rugby World Cup with Guy. In no time, I had my feet under the table, the outdoor one at first and, more intimately, the specially dedicated swimmers' one in the Café on wetter days. I was included in tips and anecdotes; trips were arranged to the play(s) I was doing; invitations made to field trips to the coast and visits to other lidos. I'd hear tales about former members of these Icicles, and about country members such as Talya. The day that David allowed me to buy my own Icicles cap was a proud one, tempered only by warnings that there were now none left for the mysterious Talya. (When I finally met her, Talya turned out to be just as beautiful and forgiving a soul as the others, of course).

Much as the comfortable swimming and good outdoor company of June through to September were stimulating, I sensed a longing among my new friends for the more challenging autumn and winter to come. I began to enjoy the anticipation of the tougher times ahead, and wonder whether or not the dipping temperature would see me off, as it does to so many. I'm a stubborn character when I choose and I thought I might continue to come in September and October through sheer belligerence, water temperature dropping as quickly as the leaves so that the end of October would see a scary 10°C. What I hadn't anticipated was that, rather than just continuing to get up each morning out of determination and under duress, the colder the pool was the more I was enjoying it. I was hooked. I'm no pharmacologist, but I suspect that the adrenaline required to overcome the fear of the cold water, followed by the wonderful mix of dopamine and endorphins produced as a result are more powerful than any drugs I ever tried or could imagine. In his excellent book, *Waterlog*, an elegy to outdoor swimming, Roger Deakin calls them 'endolphins'. That's what they feel like. A cynical psychologist might call it a polite and acceptable way to self-harm, and I couldn't deny the addictive similarity, but at least

this form has added physical benefits. I think 7–8°C is optimum for me. I'm no hero when it comes to distance or speed at that temperature; I go with the commonplace wisdom of 'a length per degree', so 7 steady lengths at 7°C is just perfect in my book.

In this, my first year, the temperature stuck around that for a welcome length of time. January 2016 eventually brought a low in the water of 4°C (0°C in the air) and I only managed 3 lengths at that. But I did. And once it was back to 5°C by February, I was elated to know I'd joined an elite band by swimming outdoors in nothing more than lycra shorts and a rubber cap through the winter drop and back again, albeit a benignly mild one. It was Maureen's first winter too. 'We had a jammy one,' she said afterwards. As the water gets below 10°C, it takes on an indescribably silky quality. Time is perceived differently and I imagine a hitherto unknown grace in my movements, a grace that's in no way apparent in warmer water as I clumsily proceed from end

to end. The other wonderful discovery is of being in nature and the weather, unfiltered and in daily doses. I'd find it amusing to chat to colleagues about their perceptions of the weather; to moans of 'God, it's rained every day this week', I'd find myself thinking, 'Actually, Tuesday was beautifully crisp and Thursday was just the finest of drizzles ...' I'd know what colours the trees at the Brixton end of the park were on any given day, and eventually how bare they'd become. I'd discover the joy of swimming in the rain, sensitive to the contrasting qualities of water of pool and precipitation.

Early spring took me to North Wales for the biggest theatre challenge of my life. Cyrano de Bergerac was a part I'd coveted for many years and I have no doubt that the physical and emotional demand of this role was made more manageable by my time at the lido and my new love of cold swimming. Without a lido in North East Wales, I found lakes, rivers and the sea as bracing substitutes in March and April. This job was truly tough. We actors

can be precious flowers at times, but I'd discovered a new hardiness, new confidence and a new gratitude for all aspects of work and play. Thrilled as I was to achieve what we did with the production and flattered by the overwhelming audience appreciation, the greatest thrill and flattery for me came on the Saturday matinée when I could look out and see a dozen or so Brockwell Icicles sat in the third row, beaming and engaged, many of whom had diverted through Chester on the way to swim in the River Dee that morning!

By early May I was back again, to that first synchro session, a brush-up lesson with Lido Mike, and to a London life I'd unknowingly yearned for: one of purpose, bond, communion, eccentricity, society, health, fun, tolerance, support, courage and hope. I'd found the Lido; I'd found outdoor swimming and with it I'd found a wonderful band of slightly unhinged fellows.

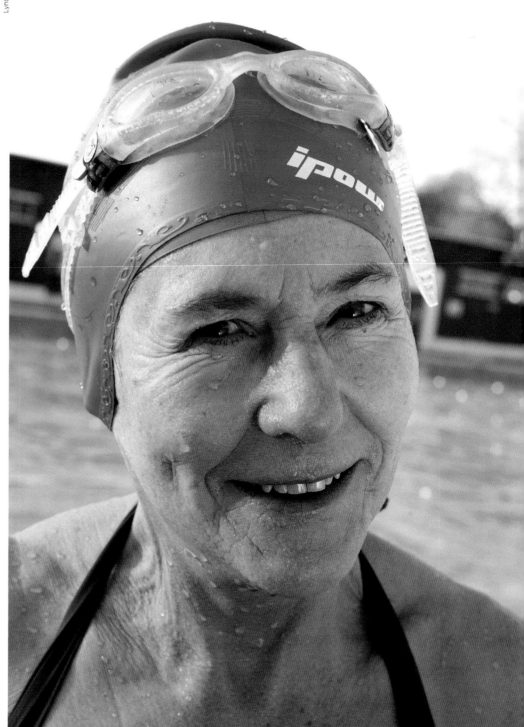

Lynda Laird

Maureen Ni Fiann
Water and light are mates, best mates

Opening the curtains, you know it's going to be a cold day – but will it be a grey day? Yes, it is.

Walking down the hill, everyone is in padded coats with hoods on their heads and with faces that look down. Everybody is buffered.

Inside your bag, the little cossie that is curled inside your towel gives you the chance to turn the grey inside out, and to walk through the looking glass.
At the lido, there is always plenty of blue. Rippling, shifting blue. Brockwell Lido, among other things, is a daily reminder of blue.

I walk in; some dive, some jump, not me, I step off planet earth. Step by step and then it's lift off – horizontal, I greet planet water and it greets me. When it is winter, you feel it in every cell, bone and centimetre of grey matter. It is ouch, for a while, but it passes.

Then the mystery begins. There are actually a few of them; I am choosing one and that is when you are in this cold blue water – you are closer to the sky.
In the water, the sky is vast. The shafts of light that are teasing their way through the grey become more visible. Water and light are mates, best mates. The light pierces the cloud successfully and is released into the water prancing, dancing and dazzling. And because of the ouch you can sense it too, in every pulse, heartbeat and centimetre of grey matter.

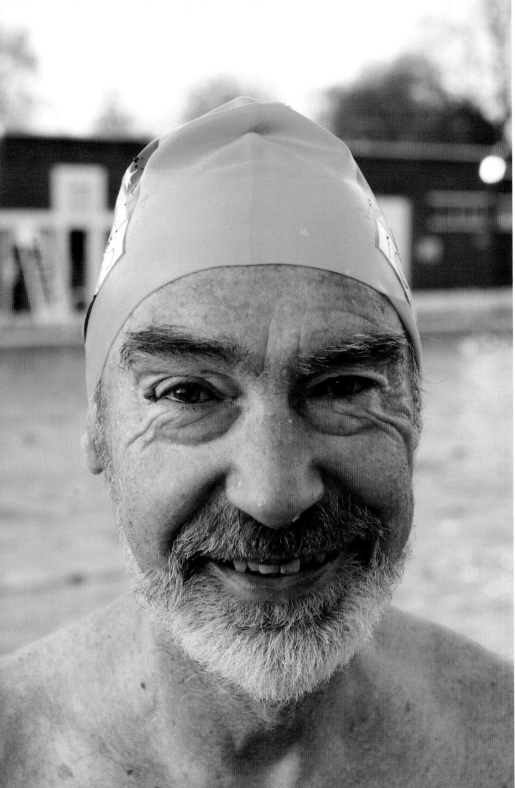
Lynda Laird

Andy Murray
I leave with a warm feeling

I first swam at the Lido occasionally in the summer in the late 1980s. Eventually, I came with wife Ros more regularly and we had summer season tickets in the Paddy and Casey era, going early in the morning and buying breakfast from the hut in the corner. Most years, the pool was open only until early September and it seemed quite cool and quite a relief to switch to indoors for the autumn and winter. One year the pool was open until the end of September and I remember everyone shivering uncontrollably after swimming at 17 degrees, which would feel warm to me now.

I have had full membership of the Lido and BLU since Fusion took over and kept up the daily summer swimming. I also run quite a bit (21 London Marathons), so don't feel the need to swim too far—10 or 12 lengths is fine for me, even when it is warm enough to do more. I always like to do the last length breaststroke, so I can look around and see the scene each day—swimmers, sky and trees. I skipped the first winter swim season, but started going early morning in the 2013–2014 winter. As soon as the temperature dipped to 15, I was in neoprene gloves, boots and t-shirt, but kept going a couple of times a week and was delighted to tick off the new months I had swum in. We were fortunate that it was a mild winter and 6 degrees was the coldest. Gradually, each winter, I have come more often and with less protection – just trunks now – I have some lovely ones from Lowie around the corner, which feature the Lido and park in their design. I try not to get too cold, perhaps cutting down the crawl to the middle third of the length between the ladders. On the darker days, the tree silhouettes can be interesting to look at. Using the spa afterwards means I leave with a warm feeling each time.

Rachael Dickens
That bright cleansing blue

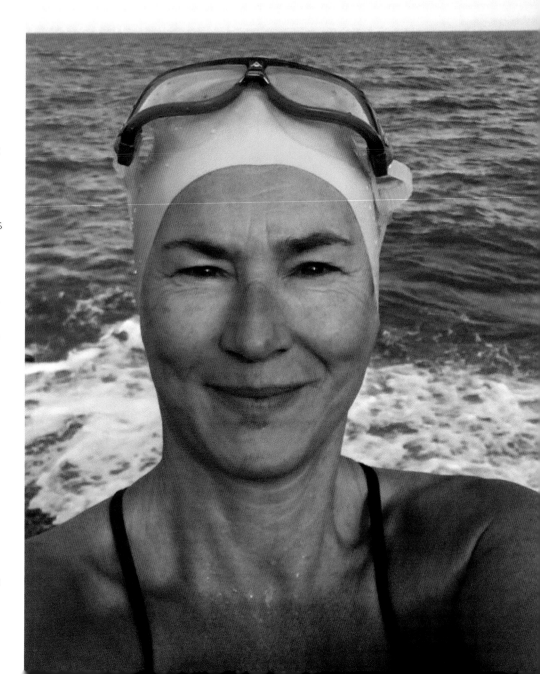

I started swimming outdoors when Crystal Palace closed for refurbishment, in 2005, I think it was. My friend from book club, Pip Tunstil, swims at Tooting and I went along with her. It was September, quite cool, I did ten lengths and was hooked. Tooting was fun, they had races every Sunday and I joined in with all that, and making cakes and a slug of whisky from the nice old Doctor whose name I forget. Anyway, I was still practising and teaching yoga then, and my swim became an amazing meditation. My mantra would silently go around in my head, keeping my stroke even and strong. It's a Kundalini chant and a very important base mantra in the Sikh Kundalini yoga school. SA, TA, NA, MA: it means infinity, life, death, rebirth.

So there I was swimming up and down and up and down ... and the weather is getting colder and colder and my mantra is growling along in my head and I swim and I swim and everything else goes! It just goes. There is nothing left to think. Nothing left to feel. And it gets colder and the mornings are dark and the pool is BIG and I'm scared every morning and have to wait till someone else arrives before I plunge myself into this Lake of a pool. Then as I continue, the images start to arrive, dreamlike, misty images just asking to be painted. And so begin the pool paintings: my head is lost while I swim, but when I get home to the studio, these paintings emerge like something out of the fog. So began a whole long series of work around cold water and pools.

I started swimming at Brockwell with Candy every now and then. I met you lot, got involved with the Icicles movement, and stayed for the winter ... then I stayed on for 5 years ... lots of work resulted ... related to the pool, to swimming, to the joy of the cold, the anticipation of walking down those beautiful steps, the thrill of the dry dive into the chilly leaf-strewn breathtaking beautiful blueness ... the 1930s architecture, the ethos of outdoor

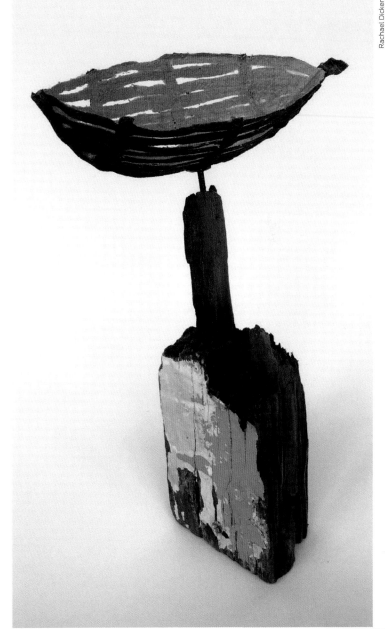

Rachael Dickens

pools in general ... healthy, no-nonsense, cracking on with life. I loved it ... had some shows and lots of fun and met new friends ... In 2014, I try to move house to get nearer the pool, the journey from Sydenham can be really long at rush hour ... an hour sometimes ... it's maddening ... London starts to be too much, the pool is the only sanctuary ... the only place I feel truly calm and happy, this can't be right. I can't afford anything nearer the lido, not with room for a studio and a dog and my kids and bike and and and ... I'm fed up with London, it's too crowded too busy too fast too noisy ... I'm single I decide to move out!

So I sell up and move to the seaside. So now I have my very own big green lido right in front of my house, it's quiet, there is rarely anyone else in it. I miss my lido chums, I miss the blue of the pool, the leaves and the ducks and the sun on the water making it sparkle and glitter like a magic potion for long life and health. It's different now ... I still swim most days: in the summer, I play for hours, diving off the groins in the clear green sea, it's washed from all around the world, it carries life and death and infinity in its very make-up ... I feel like I'm swimming in a never-ending soup of humanity, living and dying and drinking and pissing and washing and being born ... it all gets washed in and out twice a day renewed refreshed ...

It took a little while to get used to the sea. I'm still scared sometimes, I wish I could see the bottom, it gives me the creeps, but that made for some interesting work ...

Sometimes in the winter I swim at Herne Bay indoor pool, where I swim a mile with my mantra still keeping my stroke strong and even.

About three times a week all through the winter, I swim in the sea, my green lido just outside my house for a dip, or in Tankerton with new friends, 2k in the summer, 12 bays at the moment, going down to 6 then 3 as it drops ... I still love the cold water, and the sea, but I do miss that bright cleansing blue!!!

One of Rachael Dickens's sea-inspired sculptures. As here, they are often constructed of pieces of driftwood. Pebbles, shells, seaweed and plastic flotsam are also used.

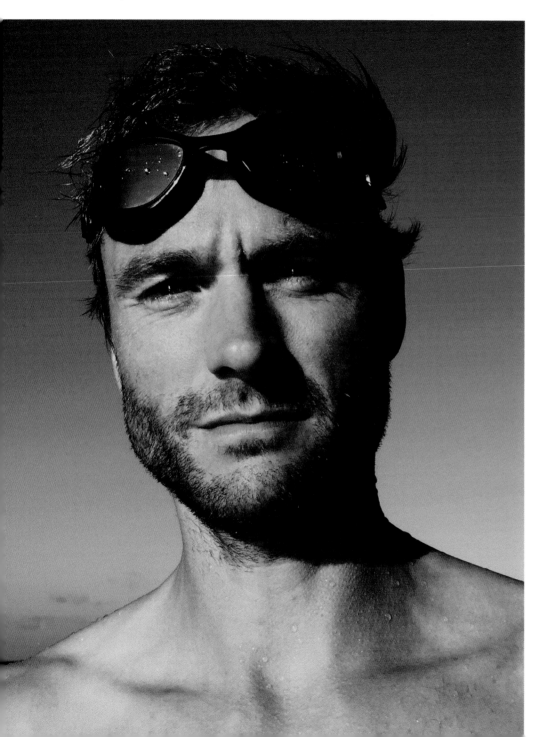

Sam Lang
Cold water swimming has re-invented swimming for me

I've always had a relationship with the water ... from swimming lessons as a kid to finding a love for surfing in my early 20s. I'm now 39, and those life responsibilities tend to get in the way of a trip to the coast.

If I'm honest, it's the ocean I truly love ... not a rectangular hole in a jam-packed city, but needs must and I have, over the years, found my fix at Brockwell Lido. When summer hits, it's the perfect 'before work city mini-break' I need ... But heading toward the winter and the decreasing daylight, I feel sad that it will be another year before I can enjoy the charm of Brixton Beach.

Until this year! This year I've decided to swim into the winter, *au naturel* (without a wetsuit) and so far it's going great. OK, so I've had to reduce my swim time and distance. I now wear a silicon swim hat and it takes a load more internal motivational speaking to get me anywhere near the pool, but cold water swimming has re-invented swimming for me. I know it's going to be cold, but I look forward to that moment when it suddenly becomes, not cold. When your skin tingles and almost burns ... making me think I've developed some 'cold-evading super power'.

There are loads of things I could list as to why I enjoy doing it, like sense of wellbeing, health, the camaraderie I share with the other swimmers, and I hope it can continue as the temperature drops ...
But most of all what I enjoy is, I feel like I shouldn't be doing it ... that I'm breaking some kind of natural law ... and that is almost the best part of all.

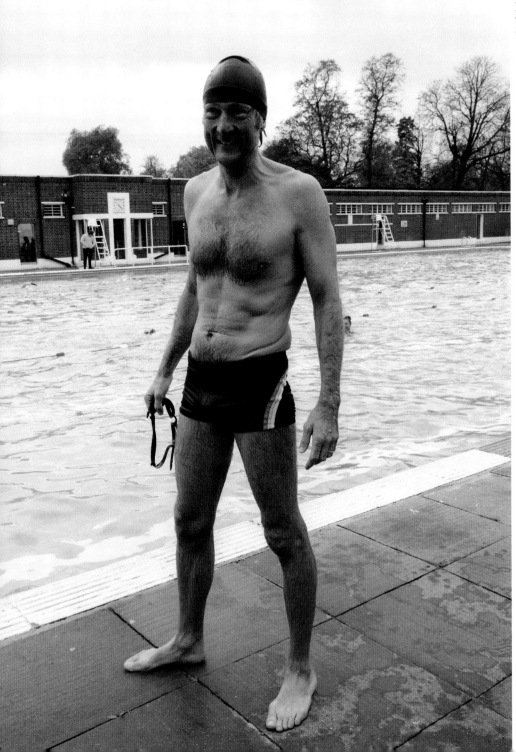

Lynda Laird

Adam Bryan
Challenging the mind as much as the body

I don't think I have any great resilience to the cold, no more than the average. I feel the winter chill like everyone else. So I don't know why I'm obsessed, slightly addicted and definitely in love with jumping into a pool of freezing water. I'm a keen swimmer, although this is about fitness, technique and a never-ending quest for a smooth and effortless style. I'll tweak this so often that I never perfect it, but not in a heated indoor pool, no way!

There is a different motivation with the cold that's about challenging the mind as much as the body and coming out the other end with a surge of endorphins and happiness. It's also about pitting myself against the weather, of being outside, and that much closer to nature, and overcoming whatever it can throw at me—in tune with the seasons and their strange and unpredictable cycle.
I do enjoy the contest—pushing myself and testing my limitations. As the pool chills from November, it's still possible to get in a decent swim; it's when it goes below 5 that it gets a little scary

and the fear can set in. There are times that I think I may have overdone it; I generally do two lengths per degree, and sometimes an extra one and then, as the goggles steam up and I can't count from ten backwards, a dreaded realisation that I have done too many.

The effort to pull myself out, my body looking red raw and a need to throw my arms in the air and wave them around in an odd rave-like warming-up dance to get through the rotten feeling. Then the rush kicks in. But most likely it is the beauty of our lovely Lido that draws me in and convinces me not to move away from the area. Sometimes it's breathtaking—the water and its many shades of blue, twinkling with the sun and reflecting its dancing rays.

So crisp and icy, gin-and-tonic fresh. It can be equally stunning at any time of day—in the dawn or dusk or even when it's overcast or raining. It's magnificently invigorating and there are many times I think I have just had the best swim ever.

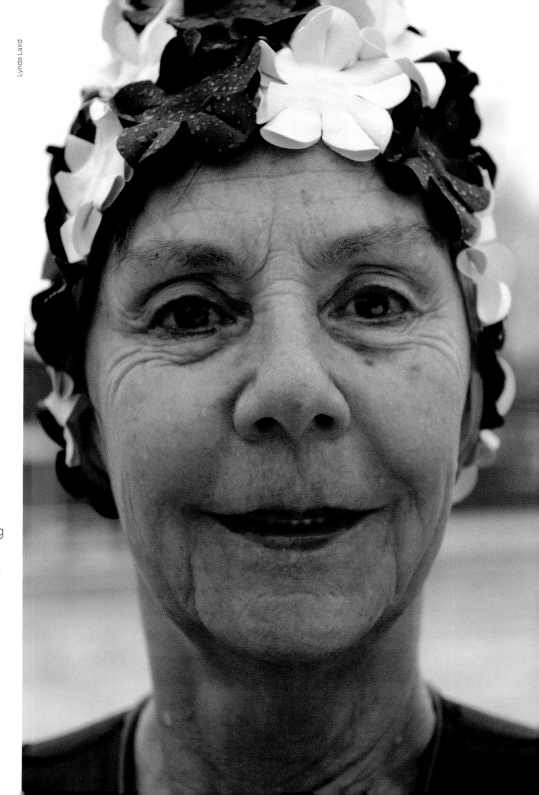

Lynda Laird

Victoria Greenwood
My oxygen remains the same

Swimming, gliding, water rolling down the body, glistening blue, turquoise, dark mysterious black. Waves chopping, sun dazzling, sky in all hues, drizzle, rain, icicles, sun, rainbows – but most of all floating silently in self thought with just lengths or time to count, contemplating ... peace.
I was born in the steamy tropics of Uganda on the banks of Lake Victoria, the provenance of my name, and obviously destined to love water. Named Little Nyanza in the hospital (Little Lake), it is said that I swam before I walked and for 60-odd years swimming has been a part of my life. I have chosen houses on the basis of their proximity to a pool, organised my daily routine around a morning dip, and ventured far and wide testing different pools and seas (and the occasional river).

An early training in the Army swimming baths in Aldershot, where a strict and vicious Major poked a stick in your arm or leg when spirits flagged, provided a steely determination to keep on going, regardless of conditions. The summers were spent at Aldershot Lido, which housed a huge blue slide and children could attend unaccompanied. My mother dropped us at the gate, only to return many hours later to exhausted, hungry children, too tired to argue. A freezing outdoor pool at boarding school where swimming was compulsory further toughened the body and provided that first sense of inhabiting one's own cocoon as the distance lengthened. The arms stretching forward, the water sliding across the body, a sense of infinity. A brief relief from the incessant noise and claustrophobia of boarding school.

At 17, I worked for a summer in Istanbul and celebrated the end of the assignment with a swim from Europe to Asia across the swirling current of the Bosphorus. It seemed nothing extraordinary, merely a teenage jaunt. A love of the sea was cemented; that ever-changing sea, dark black to turquoise green, shingle, rocks, and sandy beaches. Waves to battle in the surf from Polzeath to the freezing Atlantic of Point de la Torche in Brittany. The tepid, colourless sea of St Tropez, rocky promontories in the Western Isles or the warm

shimmering blues of the Croatian coast. There have always been islands to circumnavigate, coves to explore, new destinations to reach.
But there has always been Brockwell. I first came to Brockwell Lido as a student in 1970, biking over from Clapham Old Town or on my way back from class. In those days, we entered through the café entrance until the summer holidays, when we would prop our bikes (unlocked) on the parkside wall (now the gym) and enter through a rotating barrier where money changed hands for a basket. Women to the left, men to the right, into the large changing rooms. Cubicles lined the room; later they were painted in all colours, and three showers completely open to the area. I remember a small cracked mirror, but no hand or hair dryers. Many years later, when Casey and Paddy ruled, we sometimes entered at the front, as now, and when the crowds descended,

the summer entrance would revert to the baskets. A kindly world where rules could be thrown to the wind. A small silent community of friendship that only centred on the pool.

The lifeguards have come and gone, the management has changed, but my routine, my oxygen remains the same. That early morning light, the sun peeping overhead, the rain drizzling quietly on the head, or the crisp glisten of frost. The rainbows curving. You enter the pool, the water laps around you, arms down, and plunge forward. Above you, the trees change, bare wood, buds, leaves, bright green unfurling, colour toughens, dark green descends, autumnal colours delve deep. And the water slips and slides. And it permeates the body charging the nerves, the blood, the mind. I am ready for another day, ready for Life.

Chapter 7

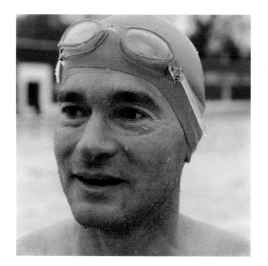

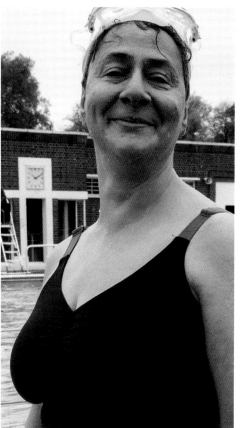

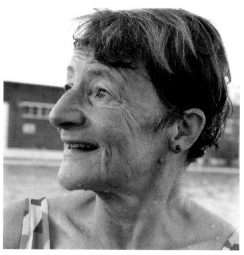

Lynda Laird

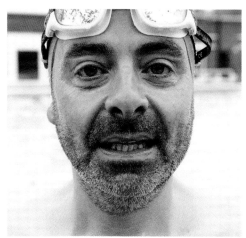

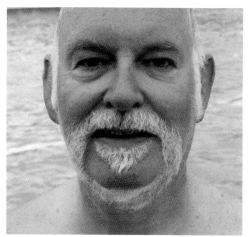

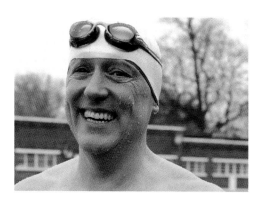

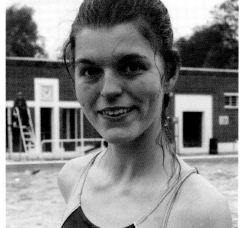

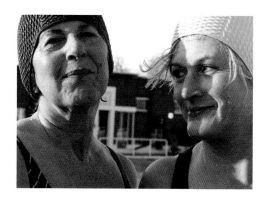

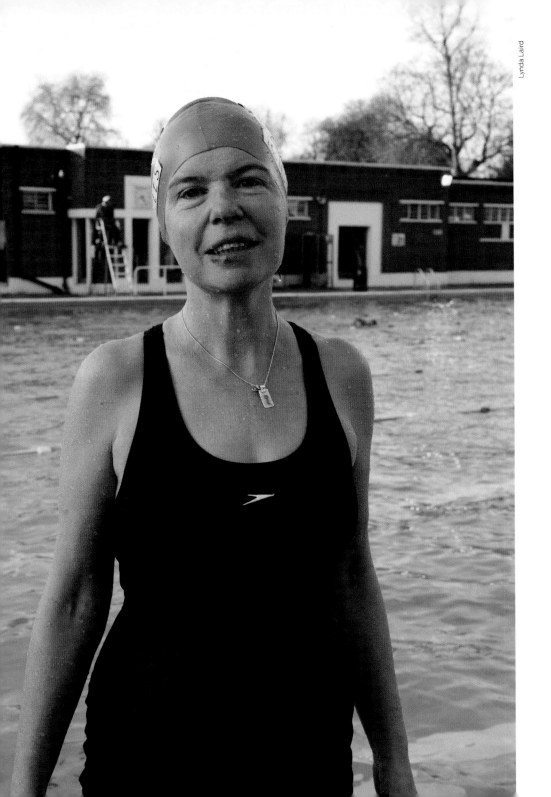
Lynda Laird

Lesley Preston
To Think I Might Never Have Known

To think I might never have known
The draw of piercing cold on skin.
That it would shock and then soothe.
And to think I might never have known
That the shifting lattice of light and liquid
That plays on the pool's sky blue floor
Would be heightened by the chill.
The quicksilver flashes on the water's steely
surface dazzle.
It is mesmerising. And now it is mine.

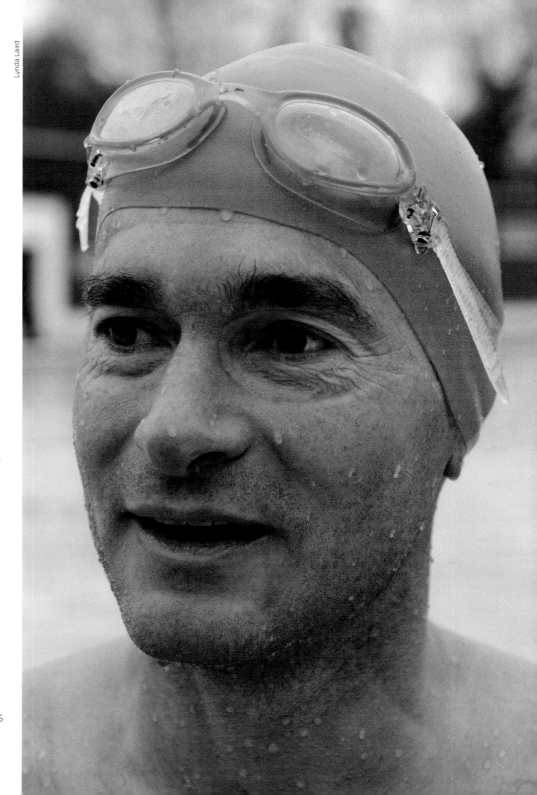

Lynda Laird

Phil Whall
Here comes the beauty

I started swimming here in October, encouraged by Angus. 'Phil, there's more magic here than in one hundred time machines,' he said. Who could resist? The water temperature was 14.0°C. That sounded cold, and my first two lengths were a big shock to my system. I was still cold at noon.
A few swims on, it's mid-November, the temperature is now 7.8°C, and I'm still going.

With the completion of that first swim, I now realise I'd accepted an unspoken challenge. Why start at all if you don't intend to continue until the arrival of Spring's warmth?
So mornings are different now. Leaving the dawn warmth of home and family, I cycle: down Sydenham Hill, Court Lane, Dulwich Village. Through slowly waking streets into misty Brockwell. I glide past early athletes, quiet walkers of dogs; the deserted children's railway. Anticipation building, mixed with nerves. Every swim is into unknown territory, as night on night the pool quietly chills.

Anoraked lifeguards already getting in place, huddling on their perches. From the classroom warmth of the changing rooms—what's the temperature?—we move outside onto the concrete apron bordering the water. Some souls dive in, seemingly fearless. I'm less brave, still learning what to expect—my first winter, and even then only in its foothills ...

OK. Down to it. The ritual makes it happen. Adjust goggles. Slip in, water to waist. I grasp the rails at the side of the pool and dip, dip, dip. Three gasps (that word seems too tame) and the shoulders are in.

No point in wasting time now. A splash of the face, and I launch. The first length passes, an adrenaline blur, the fastest length of my session, my forehead and cheek aching with anaesthetic pain. I'm already at the deep end. A pause. A couple of gasps. I made it. I made it. Press on. The third length, and I'm settling down, stretching out. Here comes the beauty. Juggling tips like spinning plates. Lengthen the body. Power from the hips. Breathe out long. Swim through a letter box. The cold retreats, time slows, marked only by strokes, breaths. Every so often, it all clicks and suddenly. I'm alone, swimming in crystal ... other swimmers close, yet a world away. Sharp bubbles of tonic surround me. I'm here. Climbing the pool rung by rung. Spiderman. I see everything—from the length of our ice-blue lagoon to pin-sharp poolfloor debris. Autumn's final leaves swaying imperceptibly below. My mind is free: people I've met. That hair clip again. The things I've done. The changing sky. Abruptly, my technique splinters—a missed breath, the line gone: it all just vanished. Focus, Phil, focus. Lengthen those arms, lessen the splash. It's humbling. There's enough time to settle again, but with every degree drop, practice time will shorten. So enjoy every second. I'm getting pins and needles in my feet now. Pushing off from the wall is painful. Almost there. Two more lengths. I can do that!
Suddenly, it's done. I drag myself out. Skin looking flushed and bruised. I hobble towards the warmth. Shaking, grinning, slightly euphoric. That first coffee will taste so good. It had better be hot. Two lengths or twenty? It doesn't matter. Everyone emerges with their own triumphs. Perhaps for veterans of several seasons these become routine pleasures. For me, every swim still an achievement. The changing room is calm, friendly. Work awaits, but not quite yet. Stories are exchanged, encouragement shared. The secret glow of the cold will last all day.
I'm a little scared of stopping now, if I'm honest. How could I even do that, though? There are more challenges to come: 6 degrees, 4 degrees and fewer all lie in wait to test me, and so I'll take each day as it comes, hoping it will all sort itself out. I'm packed for tomorrow, so lucky to have found a new adventure, and a lovely community, and all of this so close to home.

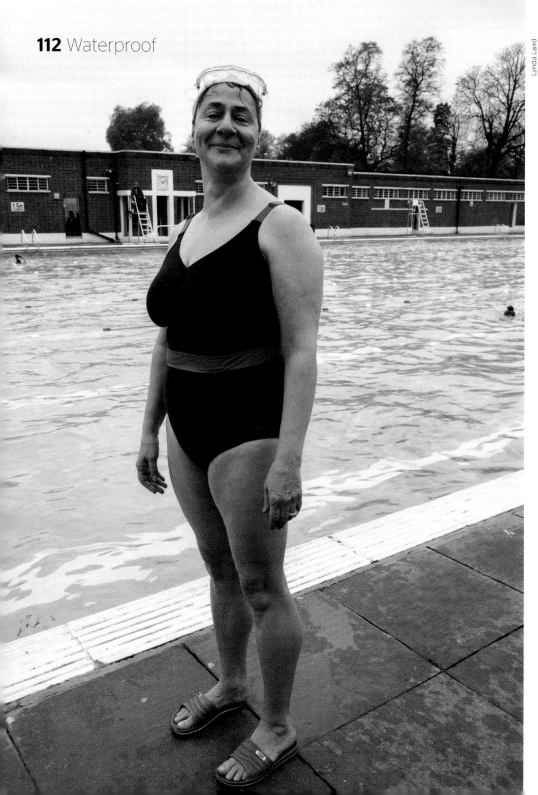

Lynda Laird

Deb Conner
Lido love

I remember very clearly at the start, the time I spent swimming in the lido was the time in the day that my body felt in a happy alliance with my head. Back then, walking to the pool was accompanied by the heaviness and fear of leaving the house. Walking back was lightness and calm, my joints were loosely connected to each other and the space around me was quiet. It was September and the water had started its slow cooling—truly the loveliest season of the year—and the sure knowledge of increasing cold gave pleasure on the day and in the anticipation.

Then the lido was not open all year. I had not embraced the delight and fear of open-water swimming and I was a cold-water novice. Clare, a hardy cold water swimmer since childhood, was hugely reassuring about the possibility of the medium. And so I was in, and I am still in. When I am away, I miss the touch of cooling water on my skin, the blue of the Lido walls and the weight of the air above.

Long ago, the roots of this love were in restoring a peaceful balance of body with mind. And since then, all this and more:

Looking out of the window in the morning, I first wonder what this cloud/rain/sun will do to the temperature of the water—whether or not there will be swimming. Then I wonder what I should wear.

Exclaiming every day, every day, 'that was lovely!' As if that day it might not have been so. The weight of evidence never so great that it took away from the joy of that moment, every moment. Swimming through the winters, we knew that we could do anything because we could do this. Relishing what comes from the nature of crawl—more completely in and of the water than above it.

A clutch of people, dearly loved and most likely unmet outside this common love of the air outside and the water underneath.

A life I would not have led. In minutes and hours in the water, at home and away, from zero to 20C, in salt, in fresh, in blue and mossy green, in dark and peaty tan, in silky and sharp, in wild and wooded, and in ice.

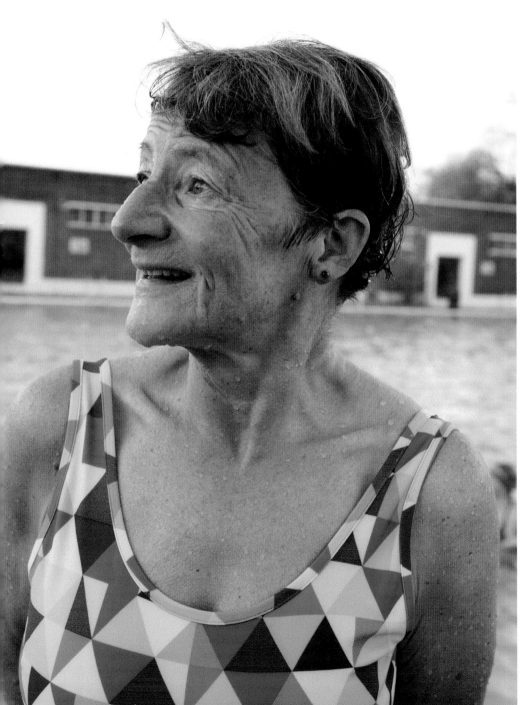

Lynda Laird

Ros Tabor
'You can never regret having a swim'

Someone once said to me, 'You can never regret having a swim' and that's very true. It's especially true with winter swimming, however long or short a time you are in the water. My shortest winter swim has been 1 length, but I still felt that it was worthwhile.

There is nothing that can beat the feeling you get when you turn round at the deep end and are greeted by full sun in your face and in the water. You push off and swim towards that lovely yellow brightness. So you have to time

it right – not too early or the sun isn't high enough, and not too late or it's too high in the sky.

Misty days, when you arrive in the park to see the mist shrouding the grass, are fantastic too.

I like to do at least one length, usually the penultimate one, on my back and look at the cloud patterns or blue skies above me.

And ... I love to share my swim with the ducks!

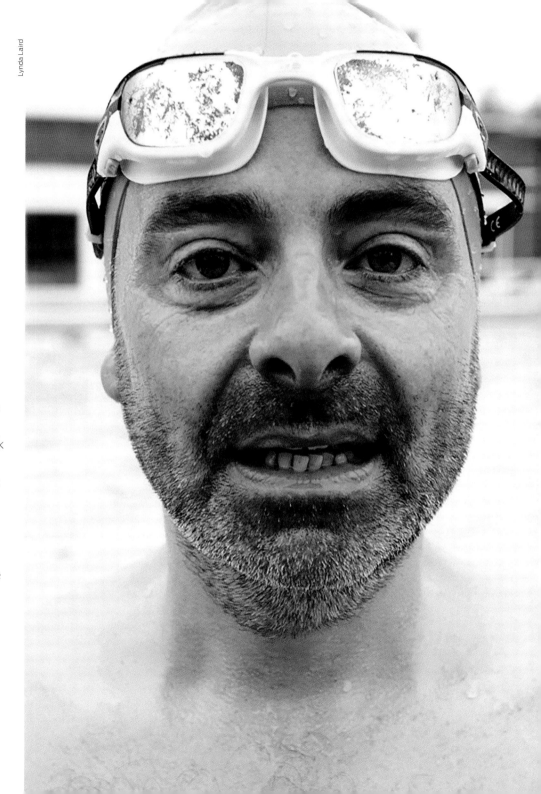

Lynda Laird

Jason Cobb
For ten minutes or so each morning in mid-winter, I can be a hero

My first experience of swimming was in an overheated municipal pool back in Nottingham. It reminded me of bath time in the family home—an uncomfortable experience, revealing body flesh in a tub so warm, you could probably boil potatoes in it. I hated it. My second experience of swimming was drifting out to sea as a young child in North Norfolk, and realising that I was in danger of drowning where they should be fishing for crabs. I loved it. The sense of freedom surrounded me as I surveyed the deepening waters.

Choppy times were ahead if I carried on with my quest to see where the water took me. The only alternative was to flap around and gain the attention of my family back on the beach.

My boyhood logic soon told me that flapping was perhaps the best thing to do. My mother caught my attention and mistook my flap for a friendly family wave. She waved back and took a photograph of me half-drowning. I confess that the choppy North Norfolk seas were only half a metre deep. This childhood memory was the start of my lifelong love affair of swimming. I have been a boy and man of water ever since. Lake Brockwell has become my North Sea substitute. I still get occasional waves from folk in the Lido Café whenever I am a little out of my depth.

I didn't fully embrace cold water swimming until very recently. The winter of 2013 was my first season of sporting the Brockwell red rash.

Pimples form all over my body from October to March. I see them as a sign of personal strength; others think that I have a low tolerance to modern life. My definition of cold water swimming has switched since three winters ago. The start of May and the opening of the Lido for the first time in the calendar was always the best day of the year.

I remember rocking up on the morning after the 2010 General Election. I hadn't slept and was without a swimming cap. The water temperature of 15 degrees caused more of a shock than the election result. Fifteen degrees and a hung Parliament would now feel like a luxury.

Yet still we return, day in, day out, all set for the ritual of the blue Brockwell experience. Make no mistake—routine is the main motivation that makes us put up with such folly first thing in the morning. Without a cold water swim and my day is lost. I need that reassurance that for ten minutes or so each morning in mid-winter, I can be a hero.

The sense of achievement is immense. It lives with me for the rest of the day, all the way through until bedtime when occasionally the tears start as I consider what I need to achieve in the morning if I don't want to accept personal failure.

It's best not to think about the process, to be honest. Just make sure that you turn up at the lovely lido, and then you will swim. I try not to contemplate what is to come as I undress and prepare for the swim.

Even the Walk of Shame past the Lido Café is an experience where swimming is the last thing on my mind. It is only when the ritual of a deep-end plunge hits me that I realise, oh—what have you just done, you fool?

And then I am away. My focus is on completing the first length. I have long since learnt not to flap like a five-year-old cast aside in North Norfolk. Breathing is everything. This needs to be controlled as you touch down for the first time in the shallow end. Rhythm and routine will carry you through the remainder of the lengths. By the end of the second length and I am giggling uncontrollably. I often wonder if the water amplifies this for my fellow cold water swimmers? I find it a genuinely funny experience each day. You are achieving something that is absolutely bonkers.

My love of cold water swimming has led me to flirt with other outdoor tarts. Tooting is too much of a big girl for me to take on. London Fields brings me out in a sweat. I once had an unfortunate experience with a dead fish at the Serpentine.

And so Lake Brockwell draws me back, day in, day out. When non-swimming friends talk about expensive foreign holidays, I just draw a complete blank. Why would you want to travel anywhere else when you have a beautiful art deco outdoor pool open all year round right on your doorstep? I do still miss North Norfolk, mind.

Lynda Laird

Jonathan Bennett
I never liked swimming in cold water

I never liked swimming in cold water. The water was always too sharp. At the first prick, my body would scream at me to get it out of there, and invariably I did. Far from relishing a winter swim, I was relieved if I made it to the end of October, when the pool closed for the winter, and would celebrate as if I had just swum the channel.

The first winter the pool stayed open, I used to scurry past, full of admiration, jealousy and ridicule for the hardy few who persisted in their madness. Occasionally, pushing my nine-month-old daughter around the weekly Parkrun in her pram, I would meet some of those (fool)hardy souls. Like Sirens, they would try and lure me in. Like Odysseus, I stuffed my ears with parsley and resisted. I wished I could have joined them, but it wasn't for me. Too cold. Too painful. Too pointless. Or maybe I knew, once lured, I would never escape.

But I felt like a coward for not giving it a go. Winter swimming felt like the kind of thing I might enjoy, no matter how little I actually wanted to do it, so the following year, I decided I had to at least try it, if only to see whether I was equal to the challenge or not. It wasn't that I wanted to swim. But I wanted to

be the kind of person who might. As if my body had got wind of my plans and wanted to prevent anything rash, just as the regular swimming season ended, a heavy cold kept me out of the water for several weeks, so I missed the incremental acclimatisation of autumn. By late November, I knew if I didn't get in soon, the challenge would prove too great and I would miss another year. If I really did want to try it out, I had no choice. It had to be now.

I trudged to the Lido with the tremulous enthusiasm of a prisoner approaching the gallows, bought my ticket and changed. The water was laughably cold. I pushed off with purpose, ignoring – or trying to – the abrupt chill, and managed a quarter of a length before the pain turned me round, screaming silently beneath the water. I couldn't do it. It hurt too much. I was getting out.

I stood in the shallows to catch my breath, and gave myself a stern talking to. Don't be so pathetic. Get back in there. This time I managed half a length. That was enough. I retreated to the changing room, my brief dalliance with winter swimming over. I had answered the question. And that answer was Absolutely Not. I was not up for winter swimming.

I lingered long under the shower, lamenting my cowardice. This is ridiculous. Can't you swim even just one length? It was no use. I would have to try again. I struggled into my trunks and marched back out, determined to reach the far end.

I marched on until the water came to my waist and I had to swim. I swam. Fighting my instincts at every stroke, I reached the end in a flailing blur of pain, and clung to the rail like a shipwrecked sailor, gasping for breath. But at least I had done it. I could retire with honour intact.

From the far end, it seemed easier to swim back than to walk, so I did. The pain seemed less now, but I was done. Not a stroke more. I was finished for the winter. I had answered the question a second time, and that answer was still Absolutely Not. I was still not up for winter swimming.

And that's where I would have left it. Except a day or two later I heard the pool calling again. Whatever it is that winter swimming does, those two lengths had done. I wanted to give it another go. See if I could swim a length without the fuss. Again I marched resolutely in. This time I managed four lengths. And that was it. I was hooked. Not so hooked that I was ready to buy a season ticket. I wasn't an addict, just an occasional user. I still thought

I could take it or leave it. So I paid my £3 for each hit, confident I could give up at any time. If that first winter was good for my health, it was ruinous for my finances. I never slipped to a pound a length, but almost. Certainly 50p. Occasionally 75. By any cost-benefit analysis, it made no sense. The following year, I bought a season ticket. The fear had returned, but I knew I could conquer it.

Now, when the pool grows warm and murky, and the lanes splash with summer swimmers, I long for the crisp, clear days of winter, the solitary swims under mournful skies when the water feels thick and syrupy, and your fingers crackle with the cold. As the temperature starts to drop and autumn takes hold, I look forward with pleasure and foreboding to the days when frost lies over the park, even to the few days when ice forms on the poolside, and slipping into the water takes on a new meaning. Encouraged by my new Lido friends, one January I swam in a fjord in northern Norway every day for a week. The air temperature was minus 13, the saltwater fjord somewhere around zero, the river beside it frozen solid. A couple of times, I bloodied my knuckles as I broke through the fine sheets of ice that floated past. Surrounded by snowy mountains, it was breath-taking in every sense,

though it felt not just foolish but properly life-threatening. Four winters on, I have learned that the first length of a cold pool is always the worst, by far. If you can manage one, you can manage several. The second will be easier, the third, yet easier. Still hard, still painful, still making you scream silently under the water with every stroke. But slightly, surreptitiously, less hard. After that, your body gets used to the assault. Your skin numbs. The pain no longer grips any one part of you, but burns your whole body like fire. By the third length, you no longer have to fight the instinct to get out immediately. Instead you can focus on how long you should endure, and what the consequences will be on the rest of your day, in numbness, shivering and bone-deep chill.

Each swim successfully swum makes the next one easier too. Easiest of all if you go every day, every two at the most, unthinking and unblinking. Any longer and the doubts start to whisper, the memory grows dark, the fear mounts: surely it was unbearable; the pain insurmountable, a repeat unthinkable. Surely this time I can't possibly survive.

The mind is a slippery fish. Best to keep it immersed at all times.
So in you go again, full of dread,

jealous of your lobster-red comrades for having swum. Trying not to think about the pain to come, just following your own personal ritual, whether you're a diver, a wader, a slipper-in. Like love, everyone comes to winter swimming differently. Like relationships, everyone has their own routines. Like life, in the end, it's just you.

You accept the pain, greet it like an inevitable acquaintance. Swim your swim. Emerge, you too, lobster-red, resplendent in your tingling badge of courage, happy that you're the one getting out, envied by your shrimp-grey colleagues as they too confront their swim.

And soon, the miracle begins, the slow onset of undefinable euphoria, the irrepressible sense of well-being that lasts all morning, sometimes all day, the addictive glow that calls you back, day after chilly day. I never liked swimming in cold water. Now I can't imagine not.

Jonathan Bennett is the author of *Around the Coast in Eighty Waves* (Sandstone Press, 2016).

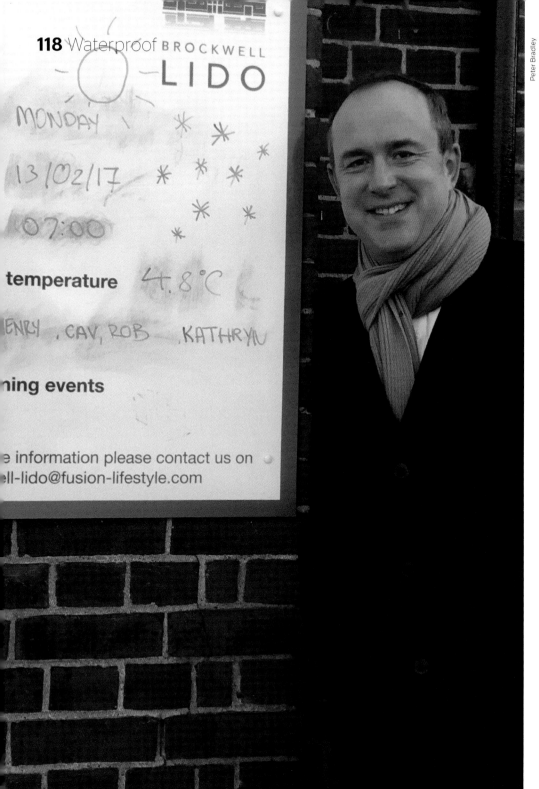

BROCKWELL LIDO

MONDAY

13/02/17

07:00

temperature 4.8°C

ENRY , CAV, ROB , KATHRYN

ning events

e information please contact us on
ell-lido@fusion-lifestyle.com

Peter Bradley

Tom Epps
Inducements

In what other sporting pursuit is carrying a little excess weight a positive advantage?

In what other sporting pursuit is a sauna encouraged and cake so celebrated?

I hope all the above are inducements to you to give it a try. If those are not enough, I would like to mention the nourishment to the soul that follows a cold water swim and the friendships that are made along the way as even more meaningful reasons to try it.

If none of that appeals, then maybe you need your spirits lifted and the cold water never fails to leave you supercharged and positive.

So I hope you will join us winter swimmers and enjoy all that winter swimming has to offer.

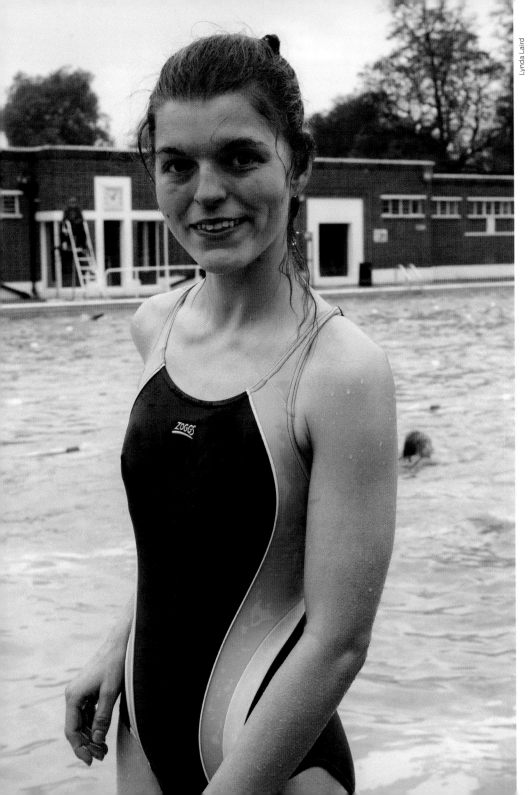

Lynda Laird

Jess Blake
It's just you and the water now

I've only been swimming here since March, but I'm hooked!

The camaraderie of cold water is amazing. I've only ever experienced anything like it before at raves. You turn up with the heat of a day's work or the fog of the morning hanging over you. You might not say much while you're peeling back the layers and getting into your cozzie. Hat on, goggles in hand, you step out of the cosy confines of the changing room. That initial bite of wind as you head poolside is the worst bit over and your skin begins to tingle with anticipation.

Jump in. It's never as bad as you fear, in fact it's lovely. And it gets more lovely as you swim, as you stretch, as you move with your breath. You feel the heat lifting from your armpits and any aches disappear along with your sense of skin. You are dissolved in this pool. Anxieties might swell up as it's just you and the water now, but then you look up at the sky and the clouds and the sun bursting over the trees, or the birds and aeroplanes passing over and you remember that the world is a wonderful, beautiful place and what an amazing thing it is to be part of it.

You come out of the water fresh but strangely warm and wow! the changing room is suddenly full of chatter and smiles. We've all had our private moment at Brockwell, but at the same time there is a deep sense of connection with those we've shared it with. Cold water swimmers truly are 'all in this [lido] together'.

Angus Scott
Something enormously positive and small b brave

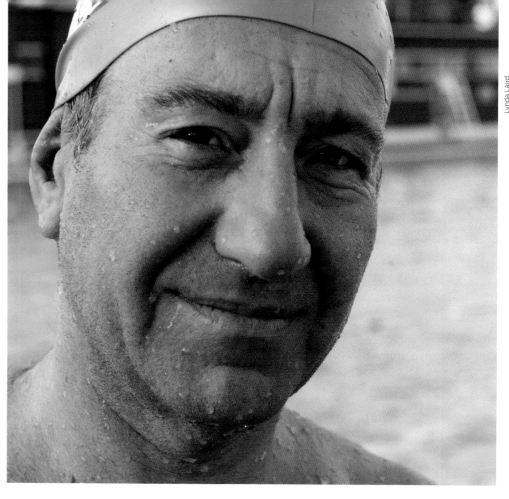

Lynda Laird

It's just nice to jump in a swimming pool isn't it, instantly surrounded by a zillion popping bubbles? Swimming in the winter is just the same, except you have the pool mainly to yourself—and fairly quickly you think, what the fuck am I doing? It's November! Then it's, hey look at that leaf! How about that? And it all started a bit earlier in the day when you woke up and thought, I've got to get down to the pool. To the vast majority, this is plainly crazy, but to a few (of us) it's like a properly strange pilgrimage, stranger even than flies to the light. Let me say I am no big fan of skiing, but I've been many times and you have to say the air is very nice; the mountain freshness of everything gets into your brain and cleanses you like a cute little fairy with a sponge. Something similar happens at the lido, in that it is such a blast out of the ordinary, the mundane; feels miles away. SO refreshing, and so friggin scary at times, and the resource is on our doorstep, our very own winter slopes, kind of, and all the pistes clear of little Tarquins. Woo hoo!
I have to say my fellow swimmers at the lido are wonderful company. None

of us particularly understands why we do this, which is probably why we're all writing these explanations. Pretty much every day we have pointless but necessary debates about the temperature, endlessly wondering whether the pool's going to be 0.1 degree colder than yesterday—it really doesn't matter, everyone's going to get in. There is surely nothing like a bit of banter with fellow certified oddballs before taking the plunge—nobody pretends it's not freezing—like we don't remember what happened yesterday ie it's cold, then it's OK, then you're done, time for medals. So you fit your hat and goggles and walk out to the chilly poolside with a rousing 'This is ground control to major Tom' in your ears. It is at this point one gets a great sense of connection to nature, specifically the weather, because somewhere in your mind there's a faint image of you explaining to the family, with your lips blue, that daddy has frozen his nuts off. In terms of the swimming itself ... obviously, it's cold, but after a bit, all the thousands of little crisis-management creatures in the body get their little emergency fires going, you

adjust, in other words, and then you are just cruising along in a beautified state, looking at leaves suspended halfway to the bottom ... or wherever. You don't spend too long in there, but 20–30 minutes is enough to give you a kind of slow burn of goodness all day. It's definitely not about trying to get better at swimming—doesn't look like it anyway—don't think that's really the point of it—it's actually more like a spa treatment. There's just something enormously positive and small b brave

about taking on the elements in the dark months and into the new year. So, having tried very hard not to be all emotional about something I love very much and without wanting to wax on, for me what it very much is about is a feeling of being lost and found at the same time. Lost in a disused Arctic disneyworld on the one hand and finding yourself floating about, oh so very happy, on the other. No better word for it. Happy. Which is why I'll do it forever. Thanks, cold water; thanks, Lido friends; thanks, Lido.

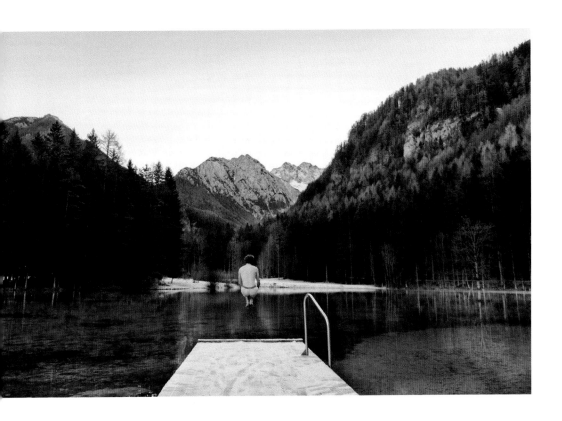

Will Kostoris
The pull of the water

Hunkered away and hidden from view
Mounted by walls, she's waiting for you

Guarded by watchmen, frozen in time
Up upon towers, line upon line

They come from afar, seeking her treasure
Dissolving each time, in liquid blue pleasure

The pull of the water, the deepest abyss
Embraces us all, in a cool tranquil kiss

Leave worries, leave woes, no stresses nor strains
A moment of calm, maintained in a lane

Peter Bradley
All the extremities, hands, feet, cock, are numb lumps

I don't know how to describe my attitude to weather at the Lido. Special to swim in the rain, diving under to watch the drops hit the surface above me, rare and more special to swim when it's snowing—the quiet of it and the brassiness of the sky it's drifting out of. Windy or still, blustery or biting, dark or searing bright, I love all weathers and don't privilege one type over another.

Today was sunny. It was special for me because I had been doing two lengths for a good while and today I managed four. I was tempted to it by the sun and by the knowledge that my fellow swimmers, particularly one hunk I'm fond of, would be piling up the lengths, so why not I? So there was the inspiration of my peers and the feeling of a personal challenge offered and met—at the end of length two, my devil whispered in my ear, 'are you really going to swim two more? Why bother, mate?'

Swimming into the sun was astounding. It was so piercingly bright, I couldn't look it in the eyes, but it sketched a sort of light show on the waves, a trembling, zig-zag pattern changing every second, that I've never noticed before. Some days, the sun prints a shocking red cloud on my retina, gorgeous, but this didn't happen today.

Because I am swimming breast stroke head up, no goggles, I can concentrate on the watery road ahead of me. The top of each ripple is printed with the fractured image of the shallow end buildings, with the trough of each ripple blank; I've noticed this shifting pattern many times and I love it. Not possible if you are doing crawl, with your head in the water looking at the bottom. Today, so strong was the sun that, as well as the ripple reflections, I caught glimpses through the surface to the bottom of the pool, where were laid the silver chasings and frettings you see every day in summer but quite rarely in winter. The whole thing—surface, bottom, swim—was an ecstatic meditation.

I turn at the shallow end, lean my back against the pool wall, and pause to relish where I am, looking at the pro-saic blue of the bottom there. I begin

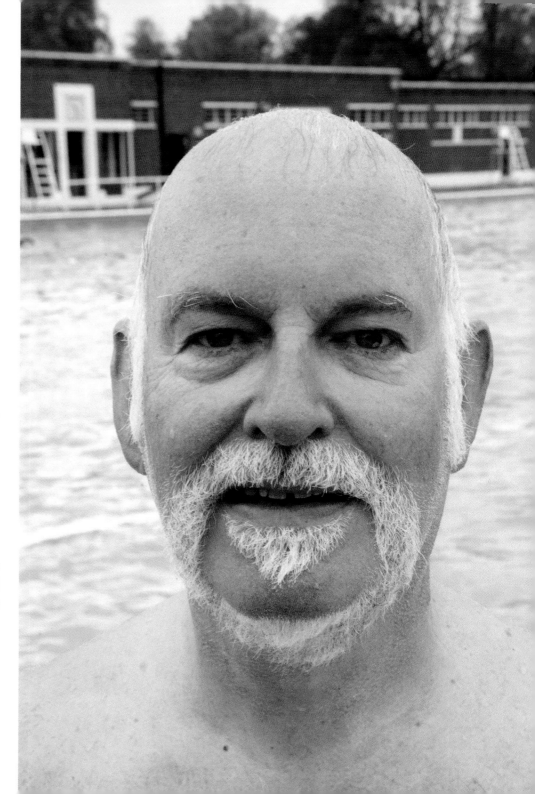

my next length with a dive, surfacing to great lightness. Because the sun is now behind me, and not in my eyes, different images present. The shattered reflections of the two white doors at the deep end quiver the whole length of the pool towards me and one ripple-wide image of the deep end after another presents itself with each stroke I make. After length 4, I haul myself out at the deep end, almost bouncing with energy.

In the shower, my hands and feet are sullen, aching blocks. I shut my eyes and my head is buzzing internally like a beehive deprived of its queen. Is this pain, this strangeness, part of what I am about, cold water swimming in Brockwell Lido? Yes.

Preliminary contemplation

Every day, something new. Today, in the shower, I realised that the shower is another form of immersion in water. We are fish; it is our element.

My mother loved swimming to the end of her days, although she came from a West of Ireland island, Inishere (now Inis Oírr), where the fishermen thought it bad luck to learn to swim: if the sea was going to get you, let it have you. And of course we live on the island of Britain, although London is far from the sea (its only fault).

Sometimes it is great to be in the changing room on my own, singing a French song as I wish, enjoying the light through the frosted-glass 1930s Crittall windows. And of course it is wonderful to be in the pool on my own; not wholly alone, as there are ever the watchful eyes of the lifeguards. But to swim alone, to have this huge space wholly to myself, that is a bliss.

Intellectually, I know the pool has to be busy in summer. Many must visit, some of whom will love it, for the lido to have a long-term future, which is what I want. But I do not like it. I do not like the changing room so full I can almost find no hook free for Bayreuth bag, or the pool so crowded I struggle to find a lane, or, when I do, get bumped into. The frenzy of it upsets me. I'm not a fast swimmer (the unkind have described my stroke as poetry in slow motion), nor a competitive one: I set myself little targets, 10 lengths, half a mile (16), or a kilometer (20) and I am pleased when, in my slow way, I meet them.

And I best like a swim when I have time to ponder things, contemplate, most of all the reflections of the surface patterns, chased fleetingly by the sun on the pool's bottom; but also, a huge, magnificent chestnut leaf, dark as sin, mysteriously suspended half-way down, responding to some strange current of its own, unaffected by us swimmers way above. And those little symbols of universal mortality, a dead bee or daddy-long-legs. And among

the living, yes, the curve of an arse or bulge of a cock or turn of a hairy thigh. All these need time and space to savour, commodities in short summer supply.

My rituals
Leaving home

First, I put on my trunks, with my swimcap/s in the left pocket and my goggles in the right, in my flat, which is opposite, and walk to the lido in my trunks, with nothing under my jacket/raincoat. So there's no faffing in the changing room: once I take off my jacket and shoes, I'm ready to swim. The rest of my clothes are in Bayreuth bag, as is, at the bottom, a spare towel in a black plastic bag.

Bayreuth bag

This is a strong, white, plastic carry all, with lovely broad grey straps. They were the chic accessory one year I was at the Wagner festival in Bayreuth. It's sturdy and capacious, almost everything a swimmer needs—almost, I say: it has no cover if heavy rain is about.

So, atop the spare towel at the bottom of Bayreuth bag go my socks, knickers, trousers, shirt and jumper. On top of that my little plastic bag (orange, from Yo Sushi) of swimming things: main towel (if I don't forget it), swimcap, with, in winter the skull cap

that goes under it, flip-flops, shampoo, spare plastic bags for je ne sais quoi.

Having donned my flip-flops, so essential for the brutal concrete of the flagstones in winter, I leave Bayreuth bag and my street shoes in the changing room and walk out to the lockers, where I deposit my overcoat/jacket with wallet and mobile phone, and my glasses that cost a king's ransom. I take the pound coin from the back pocket of my trunks to insert in the locker. I put on my swimcap(s), lock the locker, don the locker bracelet and walk down the café side of the pool, chatting to, or just greeting, the lifeguards en passant.

Drinking fountain

Two major rituals occur at the deep end. First, I have a trinitarian—must be my Catholic upbringing—three quaffs of water at the modest little drinking fountain against the wall. It is not original; in 1937, the plans show the drinking fountain as a freestanding column between the deep end flower beds. No other drinking fountain is marked on the plan. There was a direct bomb hit on this end of the lido in the second world war, so perhaps it went then. Anyway, the present one smacks of 1950s frugality and practicality. People pay it little heed nowadays—I love to see a damp patch around it that shows someone before me has used it—but I do so religiously, partly on the 'use it or lose it' principle. Mostly, though, being water, it is part of my approach to the water I swim in. Part of me also genuinely wants to wet my whistle, before I get in. There is some sort of link between the two, but it is a mysterious one, symbolised by the number of quaffs—always three, no more, no less: 'tis an odd number, a prime number, Japanese asymmetry.

The water in the fountain tells me things. In summer, it comes out warm, which I don't like. In winter, its coldness is a harbinger of my swim. Some days, it is so cold I can barely squeeze it out into my mouth. Once or twice, the pressure is so low it barely rises to my waiting lips. On the very coldest of days, there's nothing and I am oddly bereft.

The deep end shower
My quaffs quaffed, I move to the second of my major rituals, the cold shower. It is of course cleansing and I tell myself I am being a thoughtful, dutiful pool user, showering before I swim, unlike the overwhelming majority of dirty dogs who can't be bothered. But truthfully, with Mr Prufrock, I say, 'That is not what I meant at all. That is not it at all.' The chief purpose of the cold shower is not cleansing, it is, by its brutality, to so bludgeon my body that I am able to enter the water the way I

want to—diving in at the deep end. Not for me the slow, tentative wading in at the shallow end, too slow, too much time to haver, to reconsider. I want a fait accompli, to plunge in *in medias res*, head first, without possibility of reprieve. In a twinkling, I want to be wholly surrounded by water of the coldest, cruellest hue, self-impelled slanting to the bottom, my whole body aghast, exhilarated. Other people do this without the aid of the cold shower, but I can't, I need it.

The dive
So, after my quaffs, I come to the shower head, knowing that when I touch its button, cold hell breaks loose. It hits my chest, I scrub my oxters and then turn to get a splash on my back, all I can bear, but enough to impel me to the lovely, white, serrated tiles that edge the pool, my launchpad to heaven and to hell. Armed by the cold shower, I do the rest of the business with dispatch—flip-flops off, then dive in.

After my last length, I sink to the bottom and kick off it, so I can bullet out of the water, spouting like Moby Dick. I'm now ready to leave.

Farewell to the pool
Exiting after my swim is another small ritual. I could depart by the steps, but it doesn't feel right; I feel I have

to haul myself out, one of the great logistical challenges of the modern era. Several things help here. First is the metal rail for grasping, under the lip of the pool. Next is the underwater ledge that adorns the pool a foot or so down at this end: many pools don't have such a thing. Last and not least is the buoyancy of water, which means that a 66-year-old such as I can exit with almost nonchalance, grasping the rail, using the water to boost me so I can stand up on the sub-aquatic shelf with both feet. Next, I place my right foot on dry land, steadying myself with both hands, the left clutching the edge of the pool, the thumb and first three fingers of my right spread like a sprinter's on the flagstone. I teeter, then momentum kicks in and I haul my left foot onto terra firma to join my right, a great sense of achievement. When I am all on dry land, I exhale a little 'ouf' or squeak of relief. If it's very cold, or I've done a very long swim, say half a mile (16 lengths), or a kilometer, I am sometimes a little shaky on my pins and need a moment or two to recover.

Putting on the flipflops with my toes is hard enough in summer, quite impossible in winter when I have lost sensation in my feet. I have to sit on a white plastic chair and ram them on with my numb hands. Again, flipflops are essential for me in the winter, when my poor, lifeless feet can't take the

skin-stripping concrete of the flags. Back to the fountain, where I confirm my swim is over, with another three—no more no less—quaffs.

The sound of one hand clapping
After my drink, I turn from the fountain to face the pool and perform the last of my major rituals. I raise both hands above my head and clap three times. This started in winter, first as a way of putting life and warmth into my gelid hands. It turned quickly into a way of congratulating myself on the achievement of braving the waters: bravo, Peter, I'm saying to myself, you've done x lengths. It still contains the aspects of warming and congratulation, but has morphed yet again into something spiritual: Buddhist, or Shinto, or perhaps just Bradley. In Shinto, you clap twice at the entrance of a shrine to draw the god's attention, to express joy at your presence at the shrine and to ward off evil spirits. There's a bit of all of those when I clap three times.

It is surprising how difficult it is to get in three good consecutive claps. I sometimes take five or six goes to get three good 'uns. Sometimes it is a paltry, minimal, local sound.

To get three powerful claps that ring out across the pool is a rare and wonderful achievement.

Only one person, Satchmo, a

lifeguard—those silent observers of our habits and quirks—has ever asked me why I do it. I gave him a fairly full answer, although I don't believe I used the word 'Shinto'. When my three claps ring out properly, I feel I have by my sound connected with the whole pool. Don't get me wrong, I love summer and its pool patterns, which you almost never see in winter, but there is a hubbub and tension that rarely goes away in that season. On an overcast winter's morning, with hardly anyone about, those three claps pierce the hush companionably.

Sans neoprene

If I could have my way, I would swim every day, wearing nothing more than a smile. The fish we once were wear no clothes in the water, so why should we? That being my attitude, wearing a wetsuit is the polar opposite of what I want to wear—nothing. It's bad enough to have to compromise and wear a pair of trunks—in which we in the 20th century are more Victorian than the Victorians, men at least, who often swam naked, including in the big lake in Brockwell Park, the Lido's forerunner. But most of all, and this is at the core of why I winter swim, I want no filter of neoprene between me and nature. I don't want the cold mitigated. I want it raw.

Hot shower

In the changing room in winter, I almost never have to wait for a shower when I get in from the ice cauldron. First, there's the mad stabbing of the shower buttons, to set the water as cold as it can go: even that feels hot, while the hottest setting burns the skin off you if you're fresh out of a freezing pool. For months in the winter, I am doing tiny amounts of swims, four lengths, six lengths, at the lowest temperatures, two, maybe only one. So it is not in any genuine sense exercise. Others quit the Lido when it gets to about 15 degrees and carry on through the winter doing a kilometer or even a mile a day in the steaming waters of Brixton Rec or Crystal Palace, where I am doing 200m in five minutes and spending 15 minutes in the shower afterwards. So if I am not exercising, what am I doing? I am pushing at an extreme, testing my salmon pink body against brutal nature.

Below 10C is when the Lido Café offers half-price coffee to swimmers and for me this era of 'single figures' is the true winter season. Some say you should swim 'a length for a degree' and above 10C I can more or less manage it. Below 10C, all bets are off for me, and I'm down to eight lengths or six or four.

Below 10C, apart from the ever-exhilarating dive in, I keep my head above water, only doing breaststroke. Even that doesn't save me from the bite. And each day becomes a daily measurement of my self against the cold: how much can I take? Can I do one more length? It's not about avoiding cold—I'm embracing it, after all—it's a pitting of a sentient, warm being against that cold. It is implacable, insensible to what I feel. It's a one-sided negotiation, with me the only one making the concessions; the game, how few or many I'm willing to make. At sub-10C, how far I can swim is dependent on a host of factors. Not just the temperature of the water itself, but also the air outside it, whether there's wind, or sun, or rain—lovely—or snow—lovelier. It must surely be possible for a mathematician to create some formula, a coefficient of time and temperature to calculate the ideal number of lengths. Then there's my own psychology, my mood that particular day, and my health: it's a fine judgement whether to swim through a cold, or give up for a day or two, to recover.

The number of lengths is almost without exception in twos: I dive in at the deep end, I want to get out at the deep end. I certainly don't want to get out at the shallow end and have to trudge barefoot on scarifying cement to collect my flipflops. Only at the very lowest temperatures—2 or 3 degrees, which I've hardly ever swum at—would I countenance doing only one length, or three.

At such low temperatures, going up by two lengths is a big ask—a hundred extra metres at a time. It would be nice to say my calculations are always fine, that my body is so sensitive it knows just how much it can take, and in the main it does. The trouble is, extreme cold plays tricks with the brain and the willpower. It lulls, it deceives and it is imperceptible in its action, deceitful and its very coldness plays games with your mind. You think you can make it—and your bravado that makes you winter-swim in the first place says, push yourself, go for it—and you can't.

Hypothermia

Twice the consequences have been dreadful. Once, it was in Tooting Bec Lido, in the days when Brockwell didn't have seven-day winter swimming and some of us went to Tooting on the days Brockwell was closed. I had been doing eight Brockwell lengths of 50m and thought I could do four Tooting lengths of 100m, or even, 100yd. I reckoned without the fact that Tooting's vast space is always a degree or two colder than Brockwell's. I did my four Tooting lengths, cold but not impossible, I thought, went into one of its painted poolside changing cubicles and closed the door. Almost at once, I collapsed like a sack onto the concrete floor, unable to cry out or, at first, to move, and hidden from the helping world. After a bit, I was able to haul myself onto the wooden bench and I slumped against the wall, not moving for a long time. Dressing was like rending flesh.

The second time was at Brockwell, when the temperature was 5 or 6 celsius. It was one of those occasions when I would perhaps have been wiser to get out at the shallow end after length 5, but custom made me go for one more. It was the darkest of winter days, no-one about but me. I made it without incident into the changing room, not feeling different to what I usually felt. Once I got into the changing room, maybe it was the contrast in temperature, but I felt rooted to the spot, catatonic, in that I couldn't

move at all. I didn't collapse, as at Tooting. I was outwardly immovable. Internally, my head was bursting and I seemed to be observing myself from the outside. I could feel the blood rushing through my veins and actually felt I could see it even, teeming and racing all over me. It was part terrifying, part thrilling.

As at Tooting, I was alone. No one came into the changing room, no friendly face I could discuss the terror and the wonder of it with.

These two incidents are at the extreme, but the Alltag of cold water swimming is only, to use a pun, different in degree. All the extremities, hands, feet, cock, are numb lumps. I'm incapable of sliding the feet into the flipflops. I have to sit on a chair and with unresponsive hands jam

them onto unresponsive feet. I have turned a bright salmon pink.

I've never had an experience as extreme again, but every now and then I stand in the shower and feel the beginning of that high—the oddness in the head, the blood going frantic walkabout in my body.

There are hardy ones who on principle refuse to take a shower, not because they don't feel the cold, but because they don't want hot water to diminish the cold. They want to go to work all a-shiver and to feel that in their body for as long as it takes for it to dissipate. That's a bridge too far for me. After the cold, I want hot to thaw the block of ice that is my body. I start on the lowest shower setting, then over minutes bring it up to full heat, waking up bit by bit the parts

of myself, including my brain, that have shut down in the cold. It's not, like most showers, about cleansing, it's about revival, resurrection and so, on a daily basis, something special, something unique.

By Georges
Almost every time, as part of that revival, I feel impelled to sing, 99 times out of 100, one air, in French: 'Ah lève-toi, soleil', from Gounod's 1867 opera, *Roméo et Juliette*. When I first heard it sung, by the incomparable Georges Thill, in a recording from the 1930s, it pierced my heart with its loveliness and manly, Gallic charm. I don't know why it springs unbidden to my throat on winter mornings, but it does, with Roméo begging the sun: 'Pure and charming star, appear! Appear!'

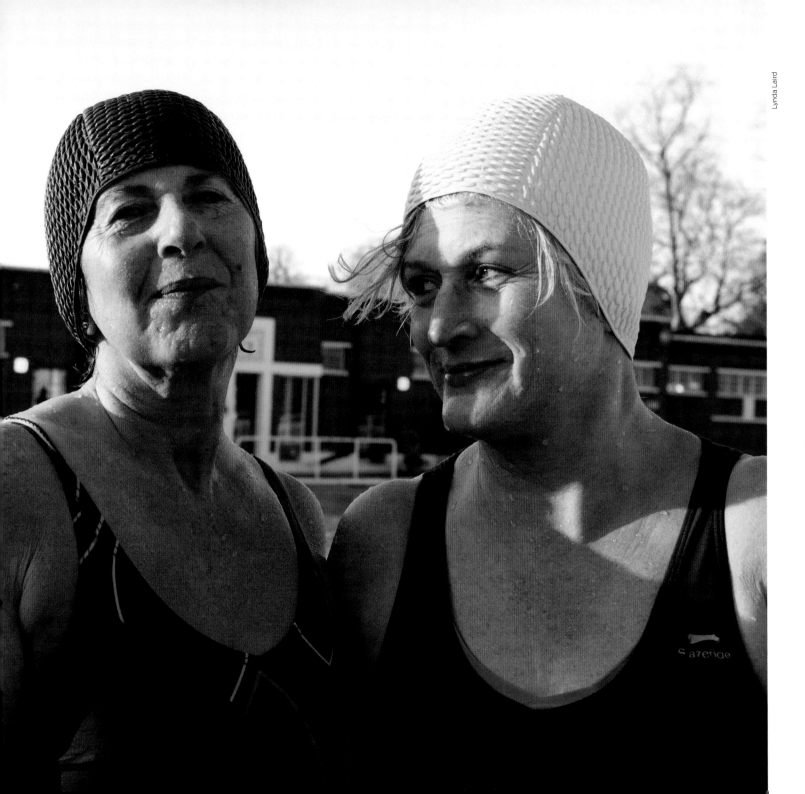

Lynda Laird

Rosemary Danielian and Miriam Ish-Horowicz
Haiku

At Brockwell Lido.
O a splash. Two friends jump in.
Keen to swim and chat.

After Bashō

**Contributors to the book were asked:
'Tell us about yourself in 25 words'**

Martin Ashworth
Difficult, reclusive pedant

Marianne Atherton
Cold water loving, ginger-haired, left-handed, cycling, vegetarian Northerner who has migrated South to enjoy the delights of Brockwell Lido.

Sara Atkinson
Happy to be living in Herne Hill and enjoying the lovely lido every day with friends and family.

Liz Barraclough
Swimmer, Atheist, Believer that we all can be better than we know. Occasional wearer of vintage swimhats; likes rivers, lakes and coldwater lidos.

Chris Bennett
Grows fruit and veg, runs in the mud, likes bikes, beer and bonfires. Three grown sons and one woman.

Jonathan Bennett
Swimmer. Surfer. Scribbler. Reluctant Londoner. Enthusiastic parent. Adequate husband. Procrastinator par excellence. Wrote about another wet adventure in *Around the Coast in Eighty Waves*.

Jess Blake
Occupational therapy student and vegan. Commonly found on two wheels or submerged in a river with a tub of peanut butter. Save the NHS!

Jonathan Blake
Once an actor now an HIV+ male who loves men, tailor/costume maker, gardener loves opera and Turkish baths an actor again LOVES coldwater swimming

Yvonne Blondell
I have swam all my life, but I am fairly new to cold water swimming. I love to sing, dance given half the chance

Peter Bradley
Second-generation Irish. Journalist. Lover of men and travel (Japan, Easter Island) and opera (Verdi and Wagner). Adore Brockwell Park and Lido. Twitter maniac.

Lisa Bretherick
Happiest in the water and on my bike. Nature liberates me, people energise and inspire me, friends and family ground me. Photographer of people.

Adam Bryan
Balearic music, natural wine, hot saunas, double dips, long socks, stripey pants, eight and bob, cary grant, la grande bellezza, crudo, negronis, coffee, always late for work, hanging out with lovely people at the lido; Ella, Wend and Gigi

Millie Burton
A work in progress…

Rosy Byatt
Homeopath and cyclist. Just moved to the seaside. Loves astrology, camping and the outdoors. Is very good at eating cake and drinking tea.

Paul Casey
London Irish, Brazilian Portuguese-speaking Hispanophile trade unionist. Owned by 3 Celia Hammond cats and married to the loveliest antique-collecting, risotto-making Italian man.

Jason Cobb
Brockwell Lido lover, Herne Hill Velodrome veteran and Surrey cricket social butterfly. Usually found walking the streets of Sunny Stockwell. *Not* an Essex Man.

Deb Conner
55, woman, mother, wife, friend, daughter, cold swimmer, walker, cook, reader, worker. Grateful for being shown more love than I might reasonably have expected.

Andrew Corrigan
The flipbook star …

Rosemary Danielian
Armenian English. Girl from the North Country now become Southern Woman. Fortunate in family, friends, the things I've done and the places I've swum.

Noelene Dasey
Giver of gas — supervisor of sleep — Australian in exile — aspiring synchronised swimmer — hydrophile and lover of lidos

Ed Errington
Lou, Dora. Two stupid, ravenous cats. Swimming, guitars. Helps make theatre happen.

David Grafton
60% water 40% mischief

John Finlay
Tropical café veteran, practical perfectionist and occasional recluse. Curious urbanite and enthusiastic driver to beautiful places. Still expecting a true vocation to reveal itself eventually.

Mark Frost
Sometime actor, recently opened small independent interiors/antiques shop in Peckham (after cold water swimming inspiration). Love design, travel, markets, occasional yoga and Wolverhampton Wanderers.

Vanessa Gibbin
Herne Hill lover. 2 mischievous children. 1 charming partner. Sustainability marketeer, Red wine and cooking enthusiast. Passion for water sports, coffee and local community.

Victoria Greenwood
Green-fingered water baby with lifelong interest in crime and punishment. Handy with boxing glove. Worldwide cyclist. Federer fanatic. Occasional tweeter.

Tommy Hanchen
From milkman to psychotherapist and forever aspiring jazz trumpeter. No matter what the surgeons or life removes, I'll find my way back into the cold water.

Sebastian Hepher
Educationalist. Headmaster for 25 years. Born in Camberwell and Milton Road resident and lido addict for the past 20 years.

Sun Ho
Designer of this book. I love my family and am proud of my country, Singapore. Good design, carefully done, can make a difference for the better in our lives.

Miriam Ish-Horowicz
Londoner by chance, Manchester by birth, with Poland and Jerusalem mixed in. The Lido is water and sky and people to share them with.

Mike Johnstone
Founder of StreamlineSwims, aka Lido Mike, professional Level 3 swim coach / teacher at Brockwell Lido. Passionate open water swimmer and cold water enthusiast. Keen cyclist.

Sarah Johnstone
SE London mum, primary school teacher, swim/art teacher and coach with @Streamlineswims. Loves long open-water swims, winter dips and zumba at Brockwell Lido.

Fran Juckes
Mother, swimmer, teacher, carpenter, knitter, stitcher, key holder, organiser, cyclist, Londoner born on River Severn, socialist who feels guilt about all the world's wrongs.

Will Kostoris
Born and bred in the Scottish Borders on the River Tweed. Water obsessed. Swimmer, diver, fisherman, Brockwell Lido fanatic. Poet.

Valerie Lambert
Careworn, ex-pat Scot and Glasgow School of Art alumna. I enjoy Scottish sea temperatures of 6 degrees upwards, and a well-made cocktail.

Sam Lang
Reluctant city dweller who constantly craves the outdoors. Director of television, lover of red wine and a complete inability to sit still.

Tauni Lanier*
'To plunge into water, to move one's whole body, from head to toe, in its wild and graceful beauty; to twist about in its pure depths, this is for me a delight only comparable to love' (Paul Valéry, French poet/ swimming enthusiast). Potential timpanist, open water– wild swimming enthusiast, unadulterated coffee snob and a keen pogonophile.
* There's always one who breaks the 25-word limit. And don't think I haven't noticed, Mr Dave Woodhead …

Lynda Laird
Photographic artist based in St Leonards on Sea. She employs techniques, methods and materials sympathetic and relevant to the subject. She focuses on long-term bodies of work. She is photographic artist in residence at the Royal Astronomical Society.

Katie Maguire
Science editor and writer. Enjoys crosswords, puns, crochet, baking. Moomin in a former life. Met Icicle Marcus at Brockwell Lido; married September 2017.

Marcus Maguire
Cycling, running and outdoor enthusiast. Loves the sea, all food and a decent pint. Works for the NHS. A regular at Christ Church Clapham. Met Icicle Katie at Brockwell Lido; married September 2017.

Geraldine Martick
Born and bred in Brixton. Lifelong lido lover, enjoys swimming, music, dancing, reading and deadheading. Independent business owner. Three cats.

Melanie Mauthner
Translator. Joined BLU in 2001 to save the Lido, Chair of BLU (2007–2010), contributed to *Out of the Blue* and co-edited, with the late Hylda Sims, *Waterwords: Lido Poems.*

Casey McGlue
Born 'n' raised in SE London, played for Harlequins, created the original Brixton Beach, one half of Beamish & McGlue, father of 2 girls, wild swimmer, music lover.

Helen Milstein
Helen: teacher, mother, wife. Amateur singer. Cold-water swimmer of some ten years. Trying to make the most of life, after years in the wilderness.

Peretz Milstein
British Israeli. Known as Polar Bear. Enjoy good company, fresh air, cold water, cake, cheese, vodka, music, dancing and cooking. Would-be artisan.

Andy Murray
Retired local government accountant. North Londoner originally, south Londoner for 40 years. Keen runner with Dulwich runners. Interested in cinema and café breakfasts.

Maureen Ni Fiann
Relationship therapist—London Irish—mum and a nana—love people and this old world of ours—made a film about pianos.

Candida Otton
Kentish Rose. Designer. Biggest wonder in my life my daughter. Lover of water, film, travel, the sun on my face, Brockwell Lido, friends and dancing.

Nick Pecorelli
English and Italian. Espresso drinker (lots). Laugher. Fairtrade entrepreneur. Psychographic pollster. Fairbnb founder. Father of a boy who fell in happiness potion. Labour.

Lesley Preston
What do I favour? Lido swim: Brockwell; Wild swim: Loch Linnhe, Lismore. Water temp: icy; sauna temp: max.

Clare Reynolds
Paper conservator (watercolour washer), lover of crosswords, scrabble, snow, knitting, and swimming (obviously): lido, synchro, wild, lake, sea, river and even in muddy shallow bogs with the right company.

Julie Reynolds
Greedy for life, wickedly dark-humoured, outdoor-swimming Yorkshire woman. Found portal to altered consciousness in cold, blue Brockwell lido. Built for distance not speed.

Steffan Rhodri
A rarely static M4 traveller between the mountains and coasts of home and urban Brixton and the haven of the Lido. And a Welsh actor.

Mike Richardson
Lover of sweat, terrifying cold, feeding and scouring.

Chris Roberts
Writer, librarian and London Tour guide. Published collection of short stories based on bus routes: *Bus Travel in South London: Stories from the City Over the Water.*

Adam Robinson
Television man. Loves family, old friends, the mountains, the deep blue, London and Brockwell Lido (especially during the cold months!).

Angus Scott
Angus—wayward non-genius dreamer happily trapped by fate to be an average family guy who loves the cold beauty of Brockwell and this sweet thing we do.

Dawn Springett
Quiet, thinking, poetic type with a passion for cooking, crafting, creating, candid conversations and cold water swimming. Always curious, questioning, challenging and learning. Still waters.

Peter Springett
Professional copywriter, content and social media expert. Co-founder outdoor swimwear retailer, KinaMara. Cooks a mean risotto. Lives in Berlin, runs marathons, speaks French, swims often.

Ros Tabor
Hertfordshire born. Lived in Camberwell since 1977. Retired primary and special needs teacher. Runner (also swimmer, walker and cross-country skier).

Ian Thel ...
... was born in Glasgow in 1982, lived in London since 2001, and plans to retire to the coast of East Lothian.

Stephen Trowell
A swimmer, runner and temperamental pessimist. Dependent on cold water, coffee, and conversation for the burst of sunshine on a cloudy day.

Carolyn Weniz
Retired college lecturer, Wiltshire born, Brixtonian for 37 years. Feel privileged to be near the Windmill, the Rec and above all, Brockwell Park and its Lido.

Phil Whall
Imperfect specimen. Loves family, easy laughers, and question askers. Kind people too. Owns too many wires. Interests? Piano, crosswords, cycling, cooking, sleep, the Horne Section.

Michael Wharley
Northerner-turned-Brixtonite, photographer and swimmer; found mostly with camera in hand, in the drink, or with one. And then: Liverpool FC, ferrets and coffee.

Carole Woddis
Cold water swimmer at Brockwell for several seasons. Still addicted to the blue stuff. Now mid-70s and missing the thrill of it all. Looking forward to Spring renewal. Hooray for Brockwell Lido. x

Dave Woodhead
Dad: with all the inherent lightning wit, innate hipness, youthful outlook and enthusiastic embracing of modern styles, tastes and technology that the term implies ... but innumerate.

Marc Woodhead
Artist, art historian. Happiest; running Blake Fell, cycling Mont Ventoux, contemplating Fra Angelico and Samuel Palmer, drawing Rodin's feet, swimming Brockwell Lido, cooking rosemary potatoes.

Michael Wynn
Yorkshire bred. Law professor. Always outdoors (one time Lakes fell runner). Enjoy poetry and remoteness (Himalaya, Java, Yunnan). Admire Joyce, Beckett, Orwell.

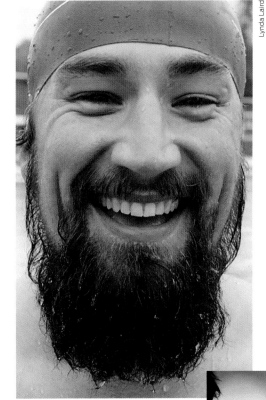
Lynda Laird

Flipbook star, Andrew Corrigan

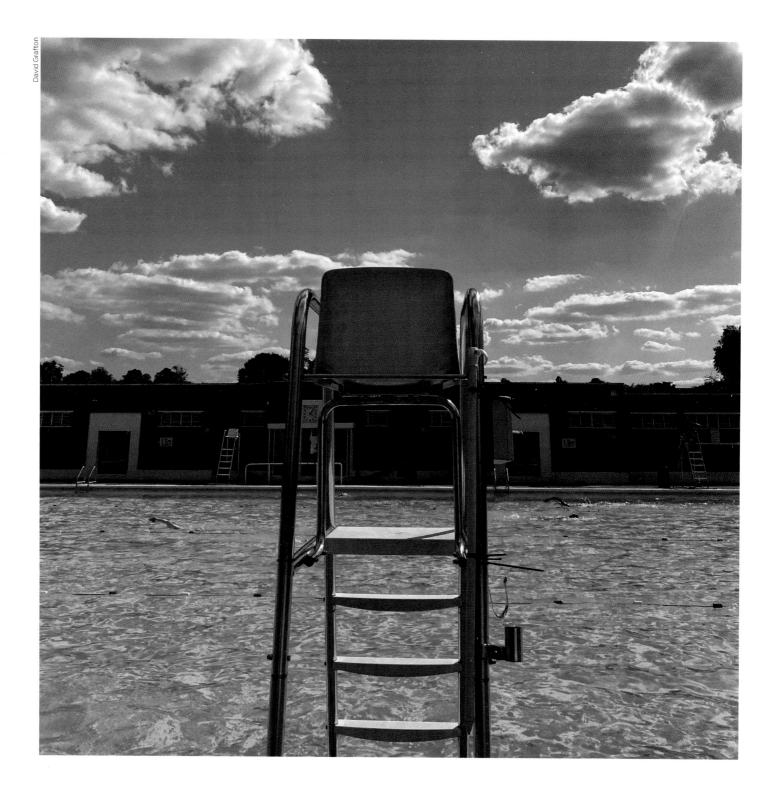

David Grafton